Acupuncture: review and analysis of reports on controlled clinical trials

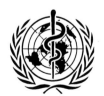

World Health Organization
Geneva
2002

WHO Library Cataloguing-in-Publication Data

Acupuncture: review and analysis of reports on controlled clinical trials.

1.Acupuncture therapy 2.Evaluation studies 3.Controlled clinical trials
4.Evidence-based medicine 5.Review literature

ISBN 92 4 154543 7   (NLM classification: WB 369)

Acknowledgements

The World Health Organization acknowledges its indebtedness to the experts who participated in the WHO Consultation on Acupuncture held in Cervia, Italy in 1996, at which the selection criteria for the data included in this publication were set. Special thanks are due to Dr Zhu-Fan Xie, Honorary Director of the Institute of Integrated Medicines, First Hospital of Beijing Medical University, China, who drafted, revised and updated this report. Further, Dr Xie made numerous Chinese language documents available in English. We also thank Dr Hongguang Dong, Geneva University Hospital, Switzerland for providing additional information.

Appreciation is extended to the Norwegian Royal Ministry of Health and Social Affairs for providing the financial support to print this review.

Contents

Introduction

Background

Over its 2500 years of development, a wealth of experience has accumulated in the practice of acupuncture, attesting to the wide range of diseases and conditions that can be effectively treated with this approach. Unlike many other traditional methods of treatment, which tend to be specific to their national or cultural context, acupuncture has been used throughout the world, particularly since the 1970s. In recognition of the increasing worldwide interest in the subject, the World Health Organization (WHO) conducted a symposium on acupuncture in June 1979 in Beijing, China. Physicians practising acupuncture in different countries were invited to identify the conditions that might benefit from this therapy. The participants drew up a list of 43 suitable diseases. However, this list of indications was not based on formal clinical trials conducted in a rigorous scientific manner, and its credibility has been questioned.

The past two decades have seen extensive studies on acupuncture, and great efforts have been made to conduct controlled clinical trials that include the use of "sham" acupuncture or "placebo" acupuncture controls. Although still limited in number because of the difficulties of carrying out such trials, convincing reports, based on sound research methodology, have been published. In addition, experimental investigations on the mechanism of acupuncture have been carried out. This research, while aimed chiefly at answering how acupuncture works, may also provide evidence in support of its effectiveness.

In 1991, a progress report on traditional medicine and modern health care was submitted by the Director-General of WHO to the Forty-fourth World Health Assembly.[1] The report pointed out that in countries where acupuncture forms part of the cultural heritage, its use in an integrated approach to modern and traditional medicine presents no difficulty. However, in countries where modern Western medicine is the foundation of health care, the ethical use of acupuncture requires objective evidence of its efficacy under controlled clinical conditions.

In 1996, a draft report on the clinical practice of acupuncture was reviewed at the WHO Consultation on Acupuncture held in Cervia, Italy. The participants recommended that WHO should revise the report, focusing on data from controlled clinical trials. This publication is the outcome of that process.

---

[1] *Traditional medicine and modern health care. Progress report by the Director-General.* Geneva, World Health Organization, 1991 (unpublished document A44/10).

Objectives

The objective of this publication is to provide a review and analysis of controlled clinical trials of acupuncture therapy, as reported in the current literature, with a view to strengthening and promoting the appropriate use of acupuncture in health care systems throughout the world. Information on the therapeutic mechanisms of acupuncture has also been incorporated.

Since the methodology of clinical research on acupuncture is still under debate, it is very difficult to evaluate acupuncture practice by any generally accepted measure. This review is limited to controlled clinical trials that were published up to 1998 (and early 1999 for some journals), in the hope that the conclusions will prove more acceptable. Such trials have only been performed for a limited number of diseases or disorders. This should not be taken to mean, however, that acupuncture treatment of diseases or disorders not mentioned here is excluded.

Use of the publication

This publication is intended to facilitate research on and the evaluation and application of acupuncture. It is hoped that it will provide a useful resource for researchers, health care providers, national health authorities and the general public.

It must be emphasized that the list of diseases, symptoms or conditions covered here is based on collected reports of clinical trials, using the descriptions given in those reports. Only national health authorities can determine the diseases, symptoms and conditions for which acupuncture treatment can be recommended.

The data in the reports analysed were not always clearly recorded. We have made every effort to interpret them accurately, in some cases maintaining the original wording in the text and summary table presented here. Research on traditional medicine, including acupuncture is by no means easy. However, researchers should be encouraged to ensure the highest possible standards of study design and reporting in future research in order to improve the evidence base in this field.

Dr Xiaorui Zhang
Acting Coordinator
Traditional Medicine (TRM)
Department of Essential Drugs
and Medicines Policy (EDM)
World Health Organization

1. General considerations

1.1 Definition

Acupuncture literally means to puncture with a needle. However, the application of needles is often used in combination with moxibustion — the burning on or over the skin of selected herbs — and may also involve the application of other kinds of stimulation to certain points. In this publication the term "acupuncture" is used in its broad sense to include traditional body needling, moxibustion, electric acupuncture (electro-acupuncture), laser acupuncture (photo-acupuncture), microsystem acupuncture such as ear (auricular), face, hand and scalp acupuncture, and acupressure (the application of pressure at selected sites).

1.2 Need for evaluation

Acupuncture originated in China many centuries ago and soon spread to Japan, the Korean peninsula and elsewhere in Asia. Acupuncture is widely used in health care systems in the countries of this region; it is officially recognized by governments and well received by the general public.

Although acupuncture was introduced to Europe as long ago as the early seventeenth century, scepticism about its effectiveness continues to exist in countries where modern Western medicine is the foundation of health care, especially in those where acupuncture has not yet been widely practised. People question whether acupuncture has a true therapeutic effect, or whether it works merely through the placebo effect, the power of suggestion, or the enthusiasm with which patients wish for a cure. There is therefore a need for scientific studies that evaluate the effectiveness of acupuncture under controlled clinical conditions.

This publication reviews selected studies on controlled clinical trials. Some of these studies have provided incontrovertible scientific evidence that acupuncture is more successful than placebo treatments in certain conditions. For example, the proportion of chronic pain relieved by acupuncture is generally in the range 55–85%, which compares favourably with that of potent drugs (morphine helps in 70% of cases) and far outweighs the placebo effect (30–35%) (1–3). In addition, the mechanisms of acupuncture analgesia have been studied extensively since the late 1970s, revealing the role of neural and humoral factors.

1.3 Evaluation methodology

Unlike the evaluation of a new drug, controlled clinical trials of acupuncture are extremely difficult to conduct, particularly if they have to be blind in design and the acupuncture has to be compared with a placebo. Various "sham" or "placebo" acupuncture procedures have been designed, but they are not easy to perform in countries such as China where acupuncture is widely used. In these countries, most patients know a great deal about acupuncture, including the special sensation that should be felt after insertion or during manipulation of the needle. Moreover, acupuncturists consider these procedures unethical because they are already convinced that acupuncture is effective. In fact, most of the placebo-controlled clinical trials have been undertaken in countries where there is scepticism about acupuncture, as well as considerable interest.

A more practical way to evaluate the therapeutic effect of acupuncture is to compare it with the effect of conventional therapy through randomized controlled trials or group studies, provided that the disease conditions before treatment are comparable across the groups, with outcome studies developed for all patients.

Because of the difficulty of ruling out the placebo effect, a comparative study with no treatment as the control may not be convincing in the evaluation of acupuncture practice. Retrospective surveys, in which the effect of acupuncture therapy is compared with past treatments, may not be of significance either, particularly if they have not been well designed. Non-comparative studies are certainly of little significance, particularly when acupuncture is used for the treatment of a self-limited disease. However, if rapid improvement can be achieved in the treatment of a long-standing, chronic disease, or if there is definite improvement in a disease that is generally recognized as intractable to conventional treatment, the effect of acupuncture should be viewed in a more favourable light, even when a well-designed, controlled study has not been carried out.

Another difficulty in evaluating acupuncture practice is that the therapeutic effect depends greatly on the proficiency of the acupuncturists—their ability and skill in selecting and locating the acupuncture points and in manipulating the needles. This may partly explain the disparities or inconsistencies in the results reported by different authors, even when their studies were carried out on equally sound methodological bases.

Evaluating acupuncture practice and arriving at generally accepted conclusions is no easy task, therefore. While effectiveness is doubtless of the utmost importance, other factors, including safety, cost, availability and the condition of local health services must also be considered. Given the same effectiveness, these other factors may lead to different evaluations of acupuncture in different countries and areas. However, conclusions are needed that apply to worldwide use, particularly for countries and areas where proper development of acupuncture practice would bring a great deal of benefit. Evaluations should not therefore be confined to those diseases for which modern conventional treatments are inadequate or ineffective.

Because of the success of surgical procedures carried out under acupuncture analgesia, the treatment of pain with acupuncture has been extensively studied. For other conditions often treated with acupuncture, there are fewer reports that have adequate methodology.

1.4   Safety

Generally speaking, acupuncture treatment is safe if it is performed properly by a well-trained practitioner. Unlike many drugs, it is non-toxic, and adverse reactions are minimal. This is probably one of the chief reasons why acupuncture is so popular in the treatment of chronic pain in many countries. As mentioned previously, acupuncture is comparable with morphine preparations in its effectiveness against chronic pain, but without the adverse effects of morphine, such as dependency.

Even if the effect of acupuncture therapy is less potent than that of conventional treatments, acupuncture may still be worth considering because of the toxicity or adverse effects of conventional treatments. For example, there are reports of controlled clinical trials showing that acupuncture is effective in the treatment of rheumatoid arthritis (4–6), although not as potent as corticosteroids. Because, unlike corticosteroids, acupuncture treatment, does not cause serious side-effects, it seems reasonable to use acupuncture for treating this condition, despite the difference in effectiveness.

1.5   Availability and practicability

The availability and practicability of acupuncture are also important factors to consider. The advantages of acupuncture are that it is simple, convenient and has few contraindications. Although the success rate of acupuncture therapy in treating kidney stones, for example, is confirmed by comparative studies with other therapies (7), it is by no means as high as that of surgical intervention. However, acupuncture treatment of kidney stones is still worth recommending because of its simplicity, which makes it more acceptable to patients.

There are also instances where acupuncture is not more practicable than conventional therapy. For example, the effectiveness of acupuncture treatment of acute bacillary dysentery has been shown to be comparable with that of furazolidone (8–10), but this is of rather academic significance because oral administration of furazolidone or other antidysenteric drugs is more convenient.

The conditions of the health service in a given country or area should also be considered in evaluating acupuncture practice. In developing countries, where medical personnel and medicines are still lacking, the need for acupuncture may be considerable and urgent; proper use of this simple and economic therapy could benefit a large number of patients. On the other hand, in developed countries, where the health system is well established, with sophisticated technology, adequate personnel and a well-equipped infrastructure, acupuncture might be considered to be of great value in only a limited number of conditions. It could still serve as a valuable alternative treatment for many diseases or conditions for which modern conventional treatments are unsuccessful. It is also valuable in situations where the patient is frightened of the potential risks or adverse effects of modern conventional treatments. In fact, in some developed countries, the diseases for which patients seek help from acupuncturists tend to be beyond the scope of orthodox medicine.

1.6   Studies on therapeutic mechanisms

Clinical evaluations indicate whether the therapy works; research on the mechanisms involved indicates how it works and can also provide important information on efficacy. Knowing that acupuncture is effective and why makes the practitioner confident in its use, and also allows the technique to be used in a more appropriate way.

The clinical evaluation may precede studies on the mechanisms, or vice versa. For acupuncture, in most instances the clinical effect has been tested first. Use of the technique may then be further expanded on the basis of the results of research on the mechanisms. For example, experimental studies of the effect of acupuncture on white blood cells led to a successful trial of the treatment of leukopenia caused by chemotherapy.

To date, modern scientific research studies have revealed the following actions of acupuncture:

- inducing analgesia

- protecting the body against infections

- regulating various physiological functions.

In reality, the first two actions can also be attributed to the regulation of physiological functions. The therapeutic effects of acupuncture are thus brought about through its regulatory actions on various systems, so that it can be regarded as a nonspecific therapy with a broad spectrum of indications, particularly helpful in functional disorders. Although it is often used as a symptomatic treatment (for pain, for instance), in many cases it actually acts on one of the pathogenic links of a disease.

Although different acupuncture points and manipulations may have an effect through different actions, the most important factor that influences the direction of action is the condition of the patient. Numerous examples reveal that the regulatory action of acupuncture is bi-directional. Acupuncture lowers the blood pressure in patients with hypertension and elevates it in patients with hypotension; increases gastric secretion in patients with hypoacidity, and decreases it in patients with hyperacidity; and normalizes intestinal motility under X-ray observation in patients with either spastic colitis or intestinal hypotonia (11). Therefore, acupuncture itself seldom makes the condition worse. In most instances, the main danger of its inappropriate application is neglecting the proper conventional treatment.

Since its therapeutic actions are achieved by mobilization of the organism's own potential, acupuncture does not produce adverse effects, as do many drug therapies. For example, when release of hydrocortisone plays an important role in the production of a therapeutic effect, the doses of this substance released by acupuncture are small and finely regulated, thereby avoiding the side-effects of hydrocortisone chemotherapy (12). On the other hand—and for the same reason—acupuncture has limitations. Even under conditions where acupuncture is indicated, it may not work if the mobilization of the individual's potential is not adequate for recovery.

1.7 Selection of clinical trial reports

In recent decades, numerous clinical trials have been reported; however, only formally published articles that meet one of the following criteria are included in this review:

- randomized controlled trials (mostly with sham acupuncture or conventional therapy as control) with an adequate number of patients observed;

- nonrandomized controlled clinical trials (mostly group comparisons) with an adequate number of patients observed and comparable conditions in the various groups prior to treatment.

In many published placebo-controlled trials, sham acupuncture was carried out by needling at incorrect, theoretically irrelevant sites. Such a control really only offers information about the most effective sites of needling, not about the specific effects of acupuncture (13). Positive results from such trials, which revealed that genuine acupuncture is superior to sham acupuncture with statistical significance, provide evidence showing the effectiveness of acupuncture treatment. On the other hand, negative results from such trials, in which both the genuine and sham acupuncture showed considerable therapeutic effects with no significant difference between them, can hardly be taken as evidence negating the effectiveness of acupuncture. In the latter case, especially in treatment of pain, most authors could only draw the conclusion that additional control studies were needed. Therefore, these reports are generally not included in this review.

The reports are first reviewed by groups of conditions for which acupuncture therapy is given (section 2). The clinical conditions covered have then been classified into four categories (section 3):

1. Diseases, symptoms or conditions for which acupuncture has been proved — through controlled trials — to be an effective treatment.

2. Diseases, symptoms or conditions for which the therapeutic effect of acupuncture has been shown, but for which further proof is needed.

3. Diseases, symptoms or conditions for which there are only individual controlled trials reporting some therapeutic effects, but for which acupuncture is worth trying because treatment by conventional and other therapies is difficult.

4. Diseases, symptoms or conditions in which acupuncture may be tried provided the practitioner has special modern medical knowledge and adequate monitoring equipment.

Section 4 provides a tabulated summary of the controlled clinical trials reviewed, giving information on the number of subjects, the study design, the type of acupuncture applied, the controls used and the results obtained.

2. Review of clinical trial reports

2.1 Pain

The effectiveness of acupuncture analgesia has already been established in controlled clinical studies. As mentioned previously, acupuncture analgesia works better than a placebo for most kinds of pain, and its effective rate in the treatment of chronic pain is comparable with that of morphine. In addition, numerous laboratory studies have provided further evidence of the efficacy of acupuncture's analgesic action as well as an explanation of the mechanism involved. In fact, the excellent analgesic effects of acupuncture have stimulated research on pain.

Because of the side-effects of long-term drug therapy for pain and the risks of dependence, acupuncture analgesia can be regarded as the method of choice for treating many chronically painful conditions.

The analgesic effect of acupuncture has also been reported for the relief of eye pain due to subconjunctival injection (14), local pain after extubation in children (15), and pain in thromboangiitis obliterans (16).

2.1.1 Head and face

The use of acupuncture for treating chronic pain of the head and face has been studied extensively. For tension headache, migraine and other kinds of headache due to a variety of causes, acupuncture has performed favourably in trials comparing it with standard therapy, sham acupuncture, or mock transcutaneous electrical nerve stimulation (TENS) (17–27). The results suggest that acupuncture could play a significant role in treating such conditions.

Chronic facial pain, including craniomandibular disorders of muscular origin, also responds well to acupuncture treatments (28–31). The effect of acupuncture is comparable with that of stomatognathic treatments for temporomandibular joint pain and dysfunction. Acupuncture may be useful as complementary therapy for this condition, as the two treatments probably have a different basis of action (2, 32).

2.1.2 Locomotor system

Chronically painful conditions of the locomotor system accompanied by restricted movements of the joints are often treated with acupuncture if surgical intervention is not necessary. Acupuncture not only alleviates pain, it also reduces muscle spasm, thereby increasing mobility. Joint damage often results from muscle malfunction, and many patients complain of arthralgia before any changes are demonstrable by X-ray. In these cases, acupuncture may bring about a permanent cure. Controlled studies on common diseases and conditions in this category have been reported by different authors, with favourable results for acupuncture treatments compared with standard therapy, delayed-treatment controls, control needling, mock TENS, or other sham acupuncture techniques. The conditions concerned include cervical spondylitis or neck pain due to other causes (33–37), periarthritis of the shoulder (38, 39) fibromyalgia (40), fasciitis (41), epicondylitis (tennis elbow) (42–44), low back pain (45–49), sciatica (50–53), osteoarthritis with knee pain (54–56), and radicular and pseudoradicular pain syndromes (57). In some reports, comparison was made between standard care and acupuncture as an adjunct to standard care. The conclusion from one such randomized controlled trial was that acupuncture is an effective and judicious adjunct to conventional care for patients with osteoarthritis of the knee (58).

Rheumatoid arthritis is a systemic disease with extra-articular manifestations in most patients. In this disease, dysfunction of the immune system plays a major role, which explains the extra-articular and articular features. Acupuncture is beneficial in the treatment of rheumatoid arthritis (4–6). While acupuncture may not improve the damage that has been done to the joints, successful pain relief has been verified in the majority of controlled studies (58). The action of acupuncture on inflammation and the dysfunctional immune system is also beneficial (5, 59).

2.1.3 Gout

In a randomized controlled trial, blood-pricking acupuncture was compared with conventional medication (allopurinol). The acupuncture group showed greater improvement than the allopurinol group. In addition, a similar reduction of uric acid levels in the blood and urine of both groups was noted (60). Plum-blossom needling (acupuncture using plum-blossom needles), together with cupping (the application to the skin of cups which are then depressurized), has been recommended for treating gouty arthritis (61).

2.1.4 Biliary and renal colic

Acupuncture is suitable for treating acute pain, provided the relief of pain will not mask the correct diagnosis, for which other treatments may be needed. Biliary and renal colic are two conditions for which acupuncture can be used not only as an analgesic but also as an antispasmodic. In controlled studies on biliary colic (62–64) and renal colic (7, 65, 66), acupuncture appears to have advantages over conventional drug treatments (such as intramuscular injection of atropine, pethidine, anisodamine (a Chinese medicine structurally related to atropine, isolated from *Anisodus tanguticus*), bucinnazine (also known as bucinperazine) or a metamizole–camylofin combination). It provides a better analgesic effect in a shorter time, without side-effects. In addition, acupuncture is effective for relieving abdominal colic, whether it occurs in acute gastroenteritis or is due to gastrointestinal spasm (67).

2.1.5 Traumatic or postoperative pain

For traumas such as sprains, acupuncture is not only useful for relieving pain without the risk of drug dependence, but may also hasten recovery by improving local circulation (68–70). Acupuncture analgesia to relieve postoperative pain is well recognized and has been confirmed in controlled studies (71–76). The first successful operation under acupuncture analgesia was a tonsillectomy. This was, in fact, inspired by the success of acupuncture in relieving post-tonsillectomy pain. Post-tonsillectomy acupuncture was re-evaluated in a controlled study in 1990, which not only showed prompt alleviation of throat pain, but also reduction in salivation and promotion of healing in the operative wound (76).

2.1.6 Dentistry

Acupuncture has been widely used in dentistry. There are reports of randomized controlled trials on the analgesic effect of acupuncture for postoperative pain from various dental procedures, including tooth extraction (77–78), pulp devitalization (79), and acute apical periodontitis (80). According to a systematic review of papers on the use of acupuncture in dentistry published between 1966 and 1996, 11 out of 15 randomized controlled studies with blind controls, appropriate statistics and sufficient follow-up showed standard acupuncture to be more effective than a placebo or sham acupuncture. It was therefore concluded that acupuncture should be considered a reasonable alternative or supplement to current dental practice as an analgesic (81). Its use in the treatment of temporomandibular dysfunction was also supported in these studies.

2.1.7 Childbirth

In childbirth, acupuncture analgesia is useful for relieving labour pain and can significantly reduce the duration of labour (82). In the case of weakened uterine contractions, acupuncture increases the activity of the uterus. Episiotomy and subsequent suturing of the perineum can also be carried out with acupuncture analgesia. In addition, the avoidance of narcotics is advantageous for newborn infants.

2.1.8 Surgery

Acupuncture analgesia has the following advantages in surgical operations. It is a very safe procedure compared with drug anaesthesia; no death has ever been reported from acupuncture analgesia. There is no adverse effect on physiological functions, whereas general anaesthesia often interferes with respiration and blood pressure, for example. There are fewer of the postoperative complications that sometimes occur after general anaesthesia, such as nausea, urinary retention, constipation, and respiratory infections. The patient remains conscious and able to talk with the medical team during the operation so that injury of the facial and recurrent laryngeal nerve can be avoided. However, remaining conscious may be a disadvantage if the patient cannot tolerate the emotional stress of the procedure.

While the benefits of acupuncture analgesia are many, the disadvantages must also be considered. The use of acupuncture is more time-consuming and in many cases may fail to bring about complete analgesia. It is often not suitable for abdominal surgery because suppression of visceral pain and muscle relaxation may be inadequate. It is not suitable in children because few children will tolerate the needling and keep still during major surgery. Also, the surgeon must be quick and deft, so that the operation can be finished before the patient develops tolerance to the needling.

In conclusion, acupuncture analgesia as an anaesthetic for surgical procedures is indicated in selected patients who show a good response to needling in the preoperative trial, particularly when they may be a poor surgical risk under conventional general anaesthesia. The use of adjuvant drugs to potentiate the effect of the acupuncture treatment is preferred. Acupuncture can also be used in combination with general anaesthesia to reduce the dosage of anaesthetic agents (83).

2.2   Infections

Acupuncture has been reported to be effective for treating acute bacillary dysentery (8–10). Its effect is comparable with that of conventional medicines such as furazolidone, but the use of acupuncture in the first line of defence against this disease is not practicable—daily performance of needling procedures is much more complicated than administering oral drug therapy. However, when no antidysenteric agent is available or the patient is allergic to antidysenteric agents, acupuncture may occasionally be used.

The results of research on the effects of acupuncture treatments that stimulate the immune system suggest that acupuncture may be of use in conjunction with other medical therapies for treating infections (84).

The effect of acupuncture on the immune system has been tested in hepatitis B virus carriers. In a comparative study, acupuncture–moxibustion is apparently superior to herbal medications in producing hepatitis B e core antibodies and reducing hepatitis B surface antigen (85). For epidemic haemorrhagic fever, compared with steroid and supportive treatments, moxibustion shortened the period of oliguria and promoted the reduction of kidney swelling (86).

Acupuncture may be useful in treating pertussis (whooping cough), by relieving cough as well as promoting a cure (87).

2.3   Neurological disorders

In the neurological field, headaches, migraines and neuralgia are the common painful conditions treated with acupuncture. Strokes and their sequelae are another major indication for acupuncture. Early treatment of paresis after stroke has proved highly effective.

Because improvement in the effects of stroke also occurs naturally, there has been some doubt about the contribution of acupuncture. In recent years, however, a number of controlled clinical evaluations have been undertaken in stroke patients. For example, in randomized controlled studies, acupuncture treatment of hemiplegia due to cerebral infarction gave better results than conventional medication (*88–93*) and physiotherapy (*94, 95*). There were also beneficial effects when acupuncture was used as a complement to rehabilitation (*96–98*).

In one study, patients with ischaemic cerebrovascular disease treated with acupuncture were compared with patients treated with conventional drugs. Nerve function, as evaluated by electroencephalographic map and somatosensory evoked potential, showed a much more marked improvement in the patients treated with acupuncture (*89*). This has been further confirmed by experimental studies. In the laboratory, a rat model of reversible middle cerebral artery occlusion was used. The somatosensory evoked potential recorded before and after the occlusion showed that electric acupuncture markedly promoted the recovery of the amplitude of the P1–N1 wave (to 58.6% in the electric acupuncture group in contrast to 25.5% in the control group after 7 days) (*93*). In addition, recent clinical studies suggest that the effectiveness of acupuncture therapy can be further promoted by using temporal acupuncture (*99, 100*).

Comparative studies have shown acupuncture treatments to be as effective for treating hemiplegia due to cerebral haemorrhage as for that due to cerebral infarction. Since early treatment with physiotherapy is unsatisfactory, it is advisable to use acupuncture as the primary treatment. Even in hemiplegia of long duration, remarkable improvements can often be achieved. Hemiplegia due to other causes, such as brain surgery, can also be improved by acupuncture (*101*). Aphasia caused by acute cerebrovascular disorders can also be treated with acupuncture (*102*).

Although acupuncture is effective for many painful conditions, there are only a few reports on post-herpetic neuralgia. Two of them were based on randomized clinical trials and provided completely opposite results (*103, 104*). Evaluation of acupuncture in the treatment of this painful condition therefore awaits further study.

Peripheral nervous disorders are often treated with acupuncture. For example, good effects for Bell's palsy have been reported in randomized controlled trials (*105, 106*). Facial spasm is another peripheral nervous disorder for which acupuncture treatment may be indicated. For this condition it has been shown that wrist–ankle acupuncture is significantly better than traditional body acupuncture (*107*).

Coma is a serious condition that can hardly be cured by acupuncture alone, but in a comparative study of two groups of patients with similar levels of coma, a significantly greater number of patients in the acupuncture group had a 50% or greater neurological recovery than those in the control group. This suggests that it is reasonable to incorporate acupuncture along with other therapeutic and supportive measures in the treatment of the comatose patient (*108*).

Insomnia can also be treated successfully with acupuncture. In randomized control trials, both auricular acupressure and auricular acupuncture had a hypnotic effect (*109, 110*).

2.4 Respiratory disorders

Acupuncture is often used in treating respiratory disorders. Allergic rhinitis is one of the major indications. In controlled studies, it has been shown that acupuncture is more effective than antihistamine drugs in the treatment of allergic rhinitis (111–115). Acupuncture's lack of side-effects is a distinct advantage in treating this condition; however, its protective effect against allergen-provoked rhinitis has not been verified (116).

The acute symptoms of tonsillitis can be effectively relieved with acupuncture (117). Since there is no information about the incidence of complications secondary to tonsillitis treated with acupuncture, in clinical practice antibiotic therapy should still be considered the treatment of choice for acute tonsillitis. For sore throats from other causes, acupuncture treatment provides definite benefits, in contrast to a placebo and acupuncture refusal (118).

Although there are conflicting results from controlled trials in treating bronchial asthma with acupuncture, the majority of the reports suggest that acupuncture is effective (119–123) and that the effect is related to the points used (122). While bronchial asthma is not cured by acupuncture, it may be substantially relieved, at least for short periods of time. The success rates quoted in the literature are 60–70%. Acupuncture has a limited role in treating acute asthmatic attacks since it is a weak bronchodilator, but it may serve as a prophylactic measure over the long term. Controlled trials have shown that acupuncture brings about modest improvement in objective parameters, with significant subjective improvement (124). Prospective randomized single-blind studies of the effects of real and sham acupuncture on exercise-induced and metacholine-induced asthma revealed that real acupuncture provided better protection than did sham acupuncture (119), but it failed to modulate the bronchial hyperreactivity to histamine (125). Corticosteroid-dependent bronchial asthma may respond better to acupuncture treatment than other types: the required dosage of corticosteroids gradually decreases during the first weeks of acupuncture treatment (126). Acupuncture may also provide symptomatic improvement in the late stages of bronchial asthma, where there are complications of disabling breathlessness due to impaired lung function (127).

2.5 Digestive disorders

Epigastric pain is a common symptom in diseases of the stomach, including peptic ulcer, acute and chronic gastritis, and gastric spasm. Acupuncture provides satisfactory relief of epigastric pain—significantly better than injections of anisodamine or morphine plus atropine, as shown in randomized controlled trials (128, 129). For gastrointestinal spasm, acupuncture is also superior to injections of atropine (130), and for gastrokinetic disturbances, the effectiveness of acupuncture is comparable with that of conventional medicine (domperidone) (131).

Another common symptom of digestive disorders is nausea and vomiting. This can be due to a disordered function of the stomach, but it is more often a symptom or sign of generalized disorders. Morning sickness, postoperative vomiting, and nausea and vomiting related to chemotherapy are frequently encountered clinically. In all these conditions, acupuncture at point *nèiguān* (PC6) seems to have a specific antiemetic effect. A recent systematic review of trials using acupuncture for antiemesis showed that 11 of 12 randomized placebo-controlled trials, involving nearly 2000 patients, supported this effect. The reviewed papers showed consistent results across different investigators, different groups of patients, and different forms of acupuncture stimulation (*132*).

Irritable colon syndrome and chronic ulcerative colitis are often difficult to treat with conventional medication. For these diseases, acupuncture may serve as a complementary or alternative therapeutic measure (*133, 134*).

Because of its analgesic effect, acupuncture can be used in endoscopic examinations, e.g. in colonoscopy. It has been reported that the effect of acupuncture to relieve pain and discomfort during the examination is comparable with that of scopolamine or pethidine with fewer side-effects (*135, 136*).

There has been extensive research on the effect of acupuncture on the digestive system, with extensive data showing its influence on the physiology of the gastrointestinal tract, including acid secretion, motility, neurohormonal changes and changes in sensory thresholds. Many of the neuroanatomic pathways of these effects have been identified in animal models (*137*).

Acupuncture shows good analgesic and antispasmodic effects on the biliary tract and, as indicated previously, can be recommended for treatment of biliary colic (*62–64*). It also has a cholagogic action, which has been demonstrated in experimental studies. In the treatment of biliary colic due to gallstones, acupuncture is not only effective for relieving the colicky pain, but is also useful for expelling the stones. Satisfactory results were reported when electric acupuncture was used in combination with oral administration of magnesium sulfate (*138*). Acupuncture treatment is also worth trying for chronic cholecystitis, even if there is acute exacerbation (*139*).

2.6 Blood disorders

Among various blood disorders, leukopenia is the most suitable for acupuncture treatment. In controlled studies, acupuncture has been shown to be more effective than batilol and/or cysteine phenylacetate in the treatment of leukopenia due to chemotherapy (*140–142*) or benzene intoxication (*143, 144*).

2.7 Urogenital disorders

Urinary retention due to functional disorders, with no organic obstruction, is often treated with acupuncture. For postpartum or postoperative urinary retention, successful micturition usually occurs immediately after one session of needling (*66, 145*). It is probably for this reason that controlled studies on this subject have been neglected. However, there has been a report of a randomized controlled trial on traumatic retention of urine, a condition more complicated than postpartum or postoperative retention. In this trial, the efficacy of acupuncture was remarkably superior to that of intramuscular injection of neostigmine bromide(*146*).

Acupuncture is not only useful for relieving renal colic, but also for expelling urinary stones (if they are not too large), because it dilates the ureter. Satisfactory results have been obtained in comparisons with conventional medication (*7*), but it is better to use acupuncture as a complementary measure in conjunction with medication or lithotripsy.

Sexual disorders are often treated with acupuncture, but conclusive results based on methodologically sound clinical studies are still lacking. Acupuncture was shown to be more effective than placebo in the treatment of non-organic male sexual dysfunction, but the improvement was not statistically significant (*147*). In another randomized controlled trial, acupuncture had a better effect than the control in the treatment of defective ejaculation (no ejaculation during intercourse) (*148*).

Acupuncture may also be helpful to patients with chronic prostatitis. As shown in a randomized controlled trial, acupuncture was superior to oral sulfamethoxazole in relieving symptoms and improving sexual function (*149*).

In women, it has been shown that acupuncture can lower urethral pressure and relieve urethral syndrome (*150, 151*). Acupuncture has also been successfully used as a prophylaxis against recurrent lower urinary tract infections (*152*).

2.8   Gynaecological and obstetric disorders

Primary dysmenorrhoea, a painful condition, is one of the major indications for acupuncture in the field of gynaecological disorders. The beneficial effect of acupuncture on this condition has been repeatedly reported in controlled trials (*153, 154*). Acupuncture relieves pain and also regulates the motility of the uterus to facilitate menstrual discharge and further alleviate the pain.

Premenstrual syndrome is characterized by cyclical mood changes and is a common condition in women of fertile age. Acupuncture seems to be helpful to patients with this syndrome. In a controlled study, the majority of the patients receiving acupuncture gained relief from symptoms and no recurrence in the six-month follow-up (*155*).

Although acupuncture was reported to be effective in the treatment of female anovular infertility (*156*), no methodologically sound, controlled trials have been reported. However, the mechanism of acupuncture in regulating abnormal function of the hypothalamic–pituitary–ovarian axis has been demonstrated in experimental studies. The data suggest that electric acupuncture with relative specificity of acupuncture points could influence some genetic expression in the brain, thereby normalizing the secretion of certain hormones, such as gonadotropin-releasing hormone, luteinizing hormone and estradiol (*157*). Acupuncture is also worth trying in the treatment of female infertility due to inflammatory obstruction of the fallopian tubes, where it seems to be superior to conventional therapy with intrauterine injection of gentamicin, chymotrypsin and dexamethasone (*158*).

Acupuncture in pregnant women should be undertaken with care. Needling at some points (namely, on the abdomen and lumbosacral region), as well as strong stimulation of certain distant points, such as *hégŭ* (LI4), *sānyīnjiāo* (SP6) and *zhìyīn* (BL67), may cause miscarriage. However, this action is useful if induction of labour is desired, such as in prolonged pregnancy; the effect is comparable with that of oxytocin by intravenous drip (*159–161*).

In early pregnancy, acupuncture at the upper limb points can be used for the prevention and treatment of morning sickness. The efficacy of acupressure at *nèiguān* (PC6) has been reported repeatedly in placebo-controlled studies (*13, 162, 163*). In order to prevent miscarriage induced by needling, acupressure is recommended for the treatment of morning sickness.

Various methods of acupuncture, such as pressure at ear points and moxibustion at *zhìyīn* (BL67) or *zúlínqì* (GB41), have been used to correct abnormal fetal position during the last three months of pregnancy. The success rates in groups treated with these methods were much higher than the occurrence of spontaneous version or in groups treated with knee-chest position or moxibustion at non-classical points (*164–167*).

Acupuncture stimulates milk secretion after childbirth and can be used to treat deficient lactation due to mental lability or depression. It has been observed that acupuncture elevates the blood prolactin level in women with deficient milk secretion after childbirth; in the majority of cases, lactation starts as the blood prolactin level increases (*168*). The clinical use of acupuncture to promote lactation has also been demonstrated in a randomized controlled study (*169*).

2.9 Cardiovascular disorders

Acupuncture is suitable for treating primary hypotension (*170, 171*) and early essential hypertension (*172–176*). It has been reported that the influence of acupuncture on hypertension might be related to its regulatory effect on the level of serum nitrogen monoxide (*177*). For primary hypotension, acupuncture seems to be more effective than general tonics. For mild and moderate essential hypertension, the hypotensive effect of acupuncture is much more potent than that of placebos and is comparable with that of certain conventional hypotensive agents. In addition, acupuncture is often effective for relieving subjective symptoms, and it has no side-effects.

Encouraging results have been reported for a number of controlled studies on the treatment of heart disease with acupuncture, particularly in psychosomatic heart disorders, such as cardiac neurosis (*178*). In coronary heart disease, acupuncture has been shown by various authors to be effective in relieving angina pectoris. Its beneficial influence has been demonstrated during coronary arteriography. Cardiological, neurophysiological and psychological observations, made in mutually independent studies, indicated that acupuncture improved the working capacity of the heart in patients with angina pectoris and activated autoregulatory cardiovascular mechanisms in healthy persons (*179*). In controlled studies, acupuncture has provided significantly greater improvement in symptoms and cardiac work capacity than either placebo (*180–182*) or conventional medication, such as glyceryl trinitrate (*183, 184*). Dilation of the coronary artery during acupuncture has been shown to be comparable with that observed during intracatheter injection of isosorbide dinitrate (*185*). In addition, acupuncture has a beneficial effect on the left ventricular function of patients with coronary heart disease, and is also more effective than nifedipine and isosorbide dinitrate (186). Nèiguān (PC6) is the point most commonly used for treating cardiac disorders. The beneficial effect of acupuncture at this point has been demonstrated by serial equilibrium radionuclide angiography (187). Acupuncture also produces haemorrheological improvement (188).

In order to avoid unexpected accidents, however, special attention should be paid to the treatment of heart disease. Acupuncturists must be able to differentiate between angina pectoris and acute myocardial infarction.

2.10 Psychiatric disorders and mental disturbances

Acupuncture is being increasingly used in psychiatric disorders. The effect of acupuncture on depression (including depressive neurosis and depression following stroke) has been documented repeatedly in controlled studies (189–194). Acupuncture is comparable with amitriptyline in the treatment of depression but has fewer side-effects. In addition, acupuncture has been found to be more effective in depressive patients with decreased excretion of 3-methyl-4-hydroxy-phenylglycol (the principal metabolite of the central neurotransmitter norepinephrine), while amitriptyline is more effective for those with inhibition in the dexamethasone suppression test (192). This suggests that these two therapies work through different mechanisms. There have also been reports that, in controlled trials of schizophrenia treatment, acupuncture might have a better effect than chlorpromazine (194, 195).

Acupuncture (auricular acupressure) is much more effective than psychotherapy in the treatment of competition stress syndrome, and is worth further study (196).

The possible use of auricular acupuncture as a treatment for opium dependence was first noted in 1973 (197). It was found that some of the patients whose postoperative pain was relieved by acupuncture were hiding a dependence on opium. In 1979, a study carried out jointly in Hong Kong and London showed that endorphin concentrations were raised by acupuncture in heroin-dependent persons, resulting in successful suppression of withdrawal symptoms. Since then, acupuncture has been used to treat dependence on a variety of substances. Many substance-abuse programmes use acupuncture as an adjunct to conventional treatment (198). Most of the reports are anecdotal, and while there have been several controlled trials (199–202), the findings have not been consistent. This entire field of research is still at an early stage, holding some promise, but requiring larger-scale and more demanding research studies (198).

Acupuncture treatment has also been used in patients who wish to give up smoking. The conclusions of different researchers are conflicting, however. Some favour acupuncture, while others dismiss its value (203–207). Probably the most convincing results are from randomized controlled trials of passive abstinence, with no suggestion or motivation to stop smoking. The patients were told they would receive acupuncture for other purposes, and they were not asked to stop smoking. A comparison of the effects of auricular acupuncture and body acupuncture was made: 70% of the auricular-acupuncture patients and 11% of those receiving body acupuncture either abstained totally from smoking or reduced the amount of consumption by half. In addition, 72% of the auricular-acupuncture patients experienced disgust at the taste of tobacco (*204*). However, in contrast, a meta-analysis of seven reports carefully selected from 16 controlled studies of smoking cessation indicated that acupuncture did not have any greater effect than the placebo (*208*).

Acupuncture has also been reported to be useful for treating alcohol recidivism. In placebo-controlled trials (with acupuncture at nonspecific points as the control), the patients in the treatment group expressed less need for alcohol than did the control patients. Patients in the treatment group also had fewer drinking episodes and admissions to a detoxification centre (*209–211*). It is interesting to note that in an experimental study on healthy volunteers, acupuncture diminished clinical alcohol intoxication by increasing the alcohol level in expired air and decreasing blood alcohol levels (*212*).

2.11 Paediatric disorders

Diarrhoea in infants and young children is still a daunting problem worldwide, particularly in developing countries. Acupuncture seems to be worth using, at least as an adjunct to conventional treatments, because it regulates intestinal function and enhances immune response without causing an imbalance in the intestinal flora as do antibiotics (*213, 214*).

Convulsions due to high fever are not infrequently encountered in infants and young children. In a controlled clinical trial, convulsions stopped two minutes after needling was started, a result superior to that of intramuscular phenobarbital injection (*215*).

Although the specific treatment for pertussis is antimicrobials, the paroxysmal coughing is usually very distressing. There has been a report that acupuncture could hasten the cure as well as relieving the cough (*87*).

There are two controlled studies indicating that acupuncture may be of some help in the treatment of Tourette syndrome in children (*216, 217*).

2.12 Disorders of the sense organs

Deaf-mute children were once extensively treated with acupuncture in China, but no methodologically sound reports have ever shown that acupuncture therapy had any real effectiveness. A recent randomized controlled clinical trial on sudden-onset deafness in adults favoured acupuncture treatment (*218*).

Acupuncture might be useful in the treatment of Ménière disease for relieving symptoms and also for reducing the frequency of attacks. It seems to be more effective than conventional drug therapy (betahistine, nicotinic acid and vitamin B_6) (*219*).

Tinnitus is often difficult to treat. Traditionally acupuncture has been believed to be effective for treating tinnitus, but only two randomized controlled clinical trials are available—with inconsistent results (*220, 221*).

Unexplained earache that is neither primary (due to ear disease) nor secondary (as referred pain), is often regarded as a manifestation of psychogenic disturbances. Acupuncture has been shown to be effective in this kind of earache in a placebo-controlled trial (222).

Acupuncture might be helpful in the treatment of simple epistaxis unassociated with generalized or local disease, but only one report of a randomized controlled clinical trial is available. This report indicates that auricular acupuncture provides a more satisfactory effect than conventional haemostatic medication (223).

2.13 Skin diseases

In some countries, many skin diseases are customarily treated with acupuncture, but very few controlled studies have been published. In a randomized controlled clinical trial on chloasma, acupuncture had a significantly better effect than vitamins C and E (224).

Some evidence favouring acupuncture treatment of herpes zoster (human (alpha) herpesvirus 3) has been reported. In a randomized controlled trial, laser acupuncture relieved pain and promoted formation of scar tissue much more quickly than treatment with polyinosinic acid (225).

Acupuncture is known to have an antipruritic effect. This has been shown experimentally in volunteers, suggesting that acupuncture could be used in clinical conditions associated with pruritus (226). Acupuncture with dermal needles (seven-star or plum-blossom needles) has traditionally been used in the treatment of neurodermatitis, but confirmation of its effect in a controlled clinical trial was only recently reported (227).

For the treatment of acne vulgaris, acupuncture, particularly ear acupuncture, is worth recommending if the reported therapeutic effects can be further proved (228, 229).

2.14 Cancers

No controlled study has been reported on the efficacy of acupuncture in the treatment of cancer itself. However, acupuncture still has uses in cancer treatments. One is to relieve cancer pain, and the other is to control the adverse reactions to radiotherapy and chemotherapy. For cancer pain, it has been reported that acupuncture provided an immediate analgesic effect similar to that of codeine and pethidine, with a more marked effect after use for two months (230). The effect was comparable with that achieved using the analgesic steps recommended by WHO (231). For radiotherapy and chemotherapy, acupuncture can greatly lessen the adverse reactions in the digestive and nervous systems, as well as providing protection against damage to haematopoiesis (232–237).

2.15 Other reports

Obesity and hyperlipaemia are becoming increasingly important medical issues. If acupuncture could help in reducing body weight and blood lipids, its clinical use could be greatly expanded. Quite a number of reports on this effect have been published, but unfortunately, almost none of them is methodologically sound. There are only two preliminary reports of randomized controlled clinical trials that can be cited here (238, 239), although criticism of the study design cannot be totally avoided.

Acupuncture may be of benefit to patients with non-insulin-dependent diabetes mellitus. Its efficacy has been shown to be superior to that of placebos and comparable with that of tolbutamide (240, 241).

Anisodamine is effective in treating excessive salivation induced by drugs (usually antipsychotics), but acupuncture seems to be more effective (242).

There are also reports on the treatment of Sjögren syndrome (sicca syndrome) (243), Raynaud syndrome (244), Stein–Leventhal syndrome (polycystic ovary syndrome) (244), and Tietze syndrome (costochondritis) (245), which indicate beneficial effects from acupuncture treatment. Since these reports have appeared only in individual papers, confirmation by further study is necessary.

3. Diseases and disorders that can be treated with acupuncture

The diseases or disorders for which acupuncture therapy has been tested in controlled clinical trials reported in the recent literature can be classified into four categories as shown below.

1. **Diseases, symptoms or conditions for which acupuncture has been proved— through controlled trials—to be an effective treatment:**

    Adverse reactions to radiotherapy and/or chemotherapy

    Allergic rhinitis (including hay fever)

    Biliary colic

    Depression (including depressive neurosis and depression following stroke)

    Dysentery, acute bacillary

    Dysmenorrhoea, primary

    Epigastralgia, acute (in peptic ulcer, acute and chronic gastritis, and gastrospasm)

    Facial pain (including craniomandibular disorders)

    Headache

    Hypertension, essential

    Hypotension, primary

    Induction of labour

    Knee pain

    Leukopenia

    Low back pain

    Malposition of fetus, correction of

    Morning sickness

    Nausea and vomiting

    Neck pain

    Pain in dentistry (including dental pain and temporomandibular dysfunction)

    Periarthritis of shoulder

    Postoperative pain

    Renal colic

    Rheumatoid arthritis

Sciatica

Sprain

Stroke

Tennis elbow

2. **Diseases, symptoms or conditions for which the therapeutic effect of acupuncture has been shown but for which further proof is needed:**

Abdominal pain (in acute gastroenteritis or due to gastrointestinal spasm)

Acne vulgaris

Alcohol dependence and detoxification

Bell's palsy

Bronchial asthma

Cancer pain

Cardiac neurosis

Cholecystitis, chronic, with acute exacerbation

Cholelithiasis

Competition stress syndrome

Craniocerebral injury, closed

Diabetes mellitus, non-insulin-dependent

Earache

Epidemic haemorrhagic fever

Epistaxis, simple (without generalized or local disease)

Eye pain due to subconjunctival injection

Female infertility

Facial spasm

Female urethral syndrome

Fibromyalgia and fasciitis

Gastrokinetic disturbance

Gouty arthritis

Hepatitis B virus carrier status

Herpes zoster (human (alpha) herpesvirus 3)

Hyperlipaemia

Hypo-ovarianism

Insomnia

Labour pain

Lactation, deficiency

Male sexual dysfunction, non-organic

Ménière disease

Neuralgia, post-herpetic

Neurodermatitis

Obesity

Opium, cocaine and heroin dependence

Osteoarthritis

Pain due to endoscopic examination

Pain in thromboangiitis obliterans

Polycystic ovary syndrome (Stein–Leventhal syndrome)

Postextubation in children

Postoperative convalescence

Premenstrual syndrome

Prostatitis, chronic

Pruritus

Radicular and pseudoradicular pain syndrome

Raynaud syndrome, primary

Recurrent lower urinary-tract infection

Reflex sympathetic dystrophy

Retention of urine, traumatic

Schizophrenia

Sialism, drug-induced

Sjögren syndrome

Sore throat (including tonsillitis)

Spine pain, acute

Stiff neck

Temporomandibular joint dysfunction

Tietze syndrome

Tobacco dependence

Tourette syndrome

Ulcerative colitis, chronic

Urolithiasis

Vascular dementia

Whooping cough (pertussis)

3. **Diseases, symptoms or conditions for which there are only individual controlled trials reporting some therapeutic effects, but for which acupuncture is worth trying because treatment by conventional and other therapies is difficult:**

Chloasma

Choroidopathy, central serous

Colour blindness

Deafness

Hypophrenia

Irritable colon syndrome

Neuropathic bladder in spinal cord injury

Pulmonary heart disease, chronic

Small airway obstruction

4. **Diseases, symptoms or conditions for which acupuncture may be tried provided the practitioner has special modern medical knowledge and adequate monitoring equipment:**

Breathlessness in chronic obstructive pulmonary disease

Coma

Convulsions in infants

Coronary heart disease (angina pectoris)

Diarrhoea in infants and young children

Encephalitis, viral, in children, late stage

Paralysis, progressive bulbar and pseudobulbar

4. Summary table of controlled clinical trials

This section provides a tabulated summary of all the controlled clinical trials reviewed for this publication. For each study, information is provided on the author(s), the year of publication, the number of subjects involved, the study design, the type of acupuncture applied, the controls used and the results obtained.

Acupuncture: review and analysis of controlled clinical trials

Condition/Study	No.	Design	Test group	Control Group	Results
Abdominal pain in acute gastroenteritis (see also Gastrointestinal spasm)					
Shu et al., 1997 (67)	25:25	Randomized controlled trial	Body acupuncture (manual)	Routine Western medication (intra-muscular atropine and promethazine)	Relief of pain was observed in: • 24 of the test group, starting 1.3 min after acupuncture • 17 of the control group, starting 11. 9 min after injection.
Acne vulgaris					
Li et al., 1998 (228)	42:42	Randomized controlled trial	Body acupuncture (manual)	Herbal medication	After 30 days of treatment, a cure was observed in: • 42.8% of the test group • 19.0% of the control group.
Wang et al., 1997 (229)	32:20	Group comparison	Auricular acupuncture	Medication (oral vitamin B_6 and antibiotics, local benzoyl peroxide ointment)	Acne disappeared after 10 days of treatment in: • 19/32 (59%) in the test group. • 7/20 (35%) in the control group.
Adverse reactions to radiotherapy and/or chemotherapy (see also Leukopenia (this includes leukopenia caused by chemotherapy); Nausea and vomiting)					
Xia et al., 1984 (237)	49:20	Randomized controlled trial	Acupuncture during radiotherapy	Radiotherapy	Acupuncture greatly lessened digestive and nervous system reactions (anorexia, nausea, vomiting, dizziness, and fatigue) due to radiotherapy and showed protection against damage to haematopoiesis.
Chen et al., 1996 (232)	44:23	Randomized controlled trial	Manual plus electric acupuncture	Western medication (metoclopramide, etc.)	Gastrointestinal reactions were cured in significantly more of the acupuncture group: • 93.2% of test group after 5.8 ± 2.7 days of treatment • 65.2% of control group after 9.4 ± 3.4 days of treatment.
Liu et al., 1998 (235)	40:40	Group comparison	Magnetic plus electric acupoint stimulation	Western medication (metoclopramide, etc.)	Acupoint stimulation therapy was comparable with intravenous metoclopramide for gastrointestinal reactions, and with dexamethasone and cysteine phenylacetate (leucogen) for leukopenia. The treatment was effective in: • 87.5% of the test group • 75.0% of the control group.
Wang et al., 1997 (236)	90	Randomized crossover study	Body acupuncture (manual)	Western medication (metoclopramide)	The treatment was effective in: • 85.6% of the test group • 61.1% of the control group.

4. Summary table of controlled clinical trials

Condition/Study	No.	Design	Test group	Control Group	Results
Li et al., 1998 (234)	22:20	Randomized controlled trial	Body acupuncture (manual)	Intravenous injection of albumin, milk fat and amino acid	Natural killer cell activity and interleukin-2 were raised in the test group, but markedly lowered in the control group. During the 3-week observation period there was: • no significant change of leukocyte and thrombocyte counts in the test group • considerable lowering of both counts in the control.

Alcohol dependence, see Dependence, alcohol

Alcohol detoxification

Thorer et al., 1996 (212)	35	Sham controlled trial	Acupuncture at two different traditional point combinations	Acupuncture at a sham point or no acupuncture	Clinical measurement using tests of equilibrium and ntation, and specific tests of metabolism and elimination of alcohol, formed the basis of the comparison. There was no difference between the sham acupuncture and no acupuncture control groups. After both traditional acupuncture point combinations, clinical effects of alcohol intoxication were minimized, while the alcohol level in the expired air increased and blood alcohol decreased.

Allergic rhinitis (including hay fever)

Chari et al., 1988 (111)	25:20	Group comparison	Acupuncture	Antihistamine (chlorphenamine)	The treatment effects were better and lasted longer in the test group and produced no adverse effects.
Jin et al., 1989 (113)	100:60	Randomized controlled trial	Acupuncture plus moxibustion	Medication (patent herbal combination: tablets containing Herba Agastachis and Flos Chrysanthemi Indici)	At follow-up 1 month after 15 days of treatment improvement was observed in: • 92/100 in the test group • 47/60 in the control group.
Huang, 1990 (112)	128:120	Randomized controlled trial	Acupuncture plus moxibustion	Antihistamine (chlorphenamine)	Treatment for 14 days was effective in: • 97% of the test group • 75.8% of the control group.
Wolkenstein et al., 1993 (247)	12:12	Randomized controlled trial	Acupuncture	Sham acupuncture	The results did not indicate a protective effect of acupuncture therapy against allergen-provoked rhinitis.

29

Acupuncture: review and analysis of controlled clinical trials

Condition/Study	No.	Design	Test group	Control Group	Results
Yu et al., 1994 (*115*)	230:30	Randomized controlled trial	Acupuncture	Antihistamine (oral astemizole plus nasal drip 1% ephedrine)	At follow-up 1 year after 4 weeks of treatment, improvement was observed in: • 94% of the test group • 76.7% of the control group.
Liu, 1995 (*114*)	50:30	Randomized controlled trial	Acupuncture at *biqiu* (located at the round prominence on the lateral mucous membrane of the lateral nasal cavity)	Nasal drip of cortisone plus ephedrine	The treatment was significantly more effective in the test group. Effective rates were: • 86.0% in the test group • 76.7% in control group.
Williamson et al., 1996 (*116*)	102	Randomized controlled trial	Acupuncture	Sham acupuncture	The therapeutic effects were similar in the two groups. In the 4-week period following the first treatment, remission of symptoms was seen in: • 39% of the test group; mean weekly symptom scores, 18.4; mean units of medication used, 4.1 • 45.2% of the control group; mean weekly symptom scores, 17.6; mean units of medication used, 5.0.

Angina pectoris, see Coronary heart disease (angina pectoris)
Aphasia due to acute cerebrovascular disorders (see also Dysphagia in pseudobulbar paralysis)

Zhang et al., 1994 (*102*)	22:22	Randomized controlled trial	Scalp acupuncture	Conventional supportive measures	Assessed by a scoring method, the therapeutic effect was much better in the test group than in the control group. Before treatment, the two groups were comparable in various respects, including causal diseases and area of lesions.

Arthritis, see Gouty arthritis; Osteoarthritis; Peri rthritis of shoulder; Rheumatoid arthritis
Asthma, see Bronchial asthma
Bell's palsy

You et al., 1993 (*106*)	25:25	Randomized controlled trial	Blood-letting acupuncture	Medication (vasodilator plus steroid, etc.)	A cure was achieved in: • 96% of the test group • 68% of the control group.
Lin, 1997 (*105*)	198:60	Group comparison	Through acupuncture (puncture of two or more adjoining points with one insertion)	Traditional acupuncture	After a 2-week treatment the cure rate was: • 90.9% in the test group • 76.7% in the control group.

Condition/Study	No.	Design	Test group	Control Group	Results
Biliary colic (see also Cholecystitis, chronic, with acute exacerbation)					
Mo, 1987 (*62*)	70:76	Group comparison	Acupuncture	Medication (injection of atropine plus pethidine)	The analgesic effect was better in the test group than in the control group.
Yang et al., 1990 (*64*)	50:50	Group comparison	Electric acupuncture	Medication (injection of anisodamine (a Chinese medicine, structurally related to atropine, isolated from *Anisodus tangutica*) plus pethidine)	Total relief of colic was achieved in 1–3 min in: • 36/50 (72%) in the test group • 12/50 (24%) in the control group. Partial relief was achieved in 5–10 min in: • 10/50 in the test group • 32/50 in the control group.
Wu et al., 1992 (*63*)	142	Group comparison	Acupuncture	Anisodamine	The treatment was effective in: • 94.3% of the test group • 80.0% of the control group.
Bladder problems, see Female urethral syndrome; Neuropathic bladder in spinal cord injury					
Breathlessness in chronic obstructive pulmonary disease					
Jobst et al., 1986 (*127*)	12:12	Randomized controlled trial	Acupuncture	Placebo acupuncture (needling at non-acupuncture "dead" points)	After 3 weeks of treatment, the test group showed greater benefit in terms of subjective scores of breathlessness and 6-min walking distance. Objective measures of lung function were unchanged in both groups.
Bronchial asthma					
Yu et al., 1976 (*123*)	20	Randomized cross-over	Acupuncture	Isoprenaline or sham acupuncture	Isoprenaline was more effective than real acupuncture. Both were more effective than sham acupuncture.
Tashkin et al., 1977 (*121*) (methacholine-induced)	12	Randomized cross-over	Acupuncture	Isoprenaline or placebo	Isoprenaline was more effective than acupuncture. Both were more effective than placebo.
Fung et al., 1986 (*119*) (exercise-induced)	19	Randomized single-blind crossover	Acupuncture	Sham acupuncture	Real acupuncture provided better protection against exercise-induced asthma than did sham acupuncture.
Tandon et al., 1989 (*125*) (histamine-induced)	16	Double-blind cross-over	Acupuncture	Acupuncture at irrelevant points	Treatment with real or placebo acupuncture failed to modulate the bronchial hyperreactivity to histamine, suggesting that a single treatment is unlikely to provide improvement in the management of acute bronchial asthma.

Acupuncture: review and analysis of controlled clinical trials

Condition/Study	No.	Design	Test group	Control Group	Results
He et al., 1994 (120)	48:48	Randomized group comparison	Laser acupuncture	Moxibustion at same points as laser acupuncture	Pulmonary ventilation indices improved in: • 33 of the test group • 20 of the control group.
Xie et al., 1996 (122)	100	Randomized controlled trial with partial crossover	Electric acupuncture at fèishū (BL 13) (n = 30)	Electric acupuncture at shàoshāng (LU11) (n =24) yújì (LU10) (n = 24), tàiyuān (LU9) (n = 30), jīngqú (LU8) (n = 28), lièquē (LU7) (n = 28) or qiūxū (GB40) (n = 24)	An anti-asthmatic effect was observed in: • 28/30 of the test group (BL 13); best immediate effect • 20/24 LU11, 22/24 LU10, 24/30 LU9, 24/28 LU8, 21/28 LU7; good effect • 4/24 GB40; least effect.
Biernacki et al., 1998 (248) (stable asthma)	23	Randomized controlled trial, double-blind crossover	Acupuncture	Sham acupuncture	There was no improvement in aspects of respiratory function measured after acupuncture or sham acupuncture. There was significant improvement in the Asthma Quality of Life Questionnaire and a parallel reduction in bronchodilators.
Bulbar paralysis after stroke (see also Dysphagia in pseudobulbar paralysis)					
Ding, 1996 (249)	120:30	Group comparison with comparable conditions	Acupuncture	Conventional Western medication (troxerutin, piracetam, Cerebrolysin: a brain peptide preparation)	Average recovery time was: • 91 (75.8%) in test group after 5.6 days of treatment • 12 (40%) in control group after 12 days of treatment.
Cancer pain					
Dang et al., 1995 (230) (stomach carcinoma)	16:16	Randomized controlled trial	Acupuncture	Western medication (codeine, pethidine)	Acupuncture treatment had: • immediate analgesic effect similar to Western medication • more marked analgesic effect than Western medication after long-term use for 2 months.
Dan et al., 1998 (231)	34:37:42	Group comparison	Body acupuncture or acupuncture plus medication	Medication (analgesic steps recommended by WHO)	An analgesic effect was observed in: • 50.0% of the medication group • 73.0% of the acupuncture group • 92.2% of acupuncture plus medication group.
Cardiac neurosis					
Zhou, 1992 (178)	30:30	Randomized controlled trial	Acupuncture at rényíng (ST9)	Medication (propranolol)	At follow-up 1 month after 10 days of treatment the therapeutic effect was better in the test group than in the control group.

Condition/Study	No.	Design	Test group	Control Group	Results
Cardiopulmonary disease, see Breathlessness in chronic obstructive pulmonary disease; Cardiac neurosis; Coronary heart disease (angina pectoris); Pulmonary heart disease, chronic					
Cerebrovascular disorders, see Aphasia due to acute cardiovascular disorders; Bulbar paralysis after stroke; Coma; Craniocerebral injury; Stroke					
Chloasma					
Luan et al., 1996 (224)	60:30	Randomized controlled trial	Auricular acupuncture plus acupressure	Vitamins C and E	After 3 months of treatment cure was achieved in: • 53.3% of the test group • 13.3% of the control group. The treatment was effective in: • 95.0% of the treatment group • 43.3% of the control group.
Cholecystitis, chronic, with acute exacerbation (see also Biliary colic)					
Gong et al., 1996 (139)	80:24	Group comparison	Body plus ear acupuncture	Conventional Western medication (unspecified)	Clinical cure (disappearance of symptoms and signs, and marked improvement of gallbladder motor function as shown by ultrasonic examination) was achieved in: • 92.5% of the test group • 32.1% of the control group.
Cholelithiasis					
Zhao et al., 1979 (138)	522:74	Group comparison	Electric acupuncture plus oral magnesium sulfate	Oral magnesium sulfate	Stones were excreted in: • 409/522 (78.4%) in the test group • 20/74 (27.4%) in the control group.
Chronic obstructive pulmonary disease, see Breathlessness in chronic obstructive pulmonary disease					
Cocaine dependence, see Dependence, opium, cocaine, heroin					
Colour blindness					
Cai, 1998 (250)	44:65: 53	Group comparison	Body acupuncture or ear acupressure	No treatment	After 1–3 courses of treatment (7–12 days each course), colour discrimination was improved: • from 0.24 to 0.46 in acupuncture group • from 0.27 to 0.52 in ear acupressure group. There was no improvement in the control group (change from 0.28 to 0.30).
Coma					
Frost, 1976 (108)	17:15	Group comparison with similar levels of coma	Acupuncture at *shéntíng* (GV24) and *shuǐgōu* (GV26)	No acupuncture	A neurological recovery of 50% or more (significant difference) was observed in: • 59% of the test group • 20% of the control group.
Competition stress syndrome					
Que et al., 1986 (196)	111:102	Randomized controlled trial	Auricular acupressure	Psychotherapy plus placebo drug	The treatment was effective in: • 92.8% of the test group • 7.8% of the control group.

Acupuncture: review and analysis of controlled clinical trials

Condition/Study	No.	Design	Test group	Control Group	Results
Convulsions in infants and young children due to high fever					
He et al., 1997 (215)	51:51	Randomized controlled trial	Acupuncture at *hégǔ* (LI4)	Intramuscular phenobarbital	Convulsions stopped 2 min after starting treatment in: • 98% of the test group • 51% of the control group.
Coronary heart disease (angina pectoris)					
Ballegaard et al., 1986 (*180*)	13:13	Randomized controlled trial	Acupuncture	Sham acupuncture (insertion of needles outside the meridians)	Cardiac work capacity (difference in pressure-rate product (dPRP)) between rest & maximum exercise & maximum PRP during exercise, was measured. No adverse effect was observed. Patients receiving active acupuncture showed significant increase in cardiac work capacity compared to those receiving sham acupuncture.
Ballegaard et al., 1990 (*181*)	24:25	Randomized controlled trial	Acupuncture	Sham acupuncture	There was a median reduction of 50% in anginal attack rate and glyceryl trinitrate consumption in both groups, with no significant difference between the groups. The increase in exercise tolerance and delay of onset of pain was significant in the test group; there were no significant changes in the control group.
Xue et al., 1992 (*186*)	42:27	Randomized controlled trial	Acupuncture	Medication (nifedipine plus isosorbide dinitrate)	Acupuncture was more effective in improving symptoms and ECG and pulse doppler ultrasonocardiography indices.
Mao et al., 1993 (*184*)	30:30	Randomized controlled trial	Acupuncture plus conventional medication	Conventional medication (glyceryl trinitrate, aspirin, calcium antagonist)	Improvement in symptoms and ECG, respectively, were observed in: • 85.7% and 69% of the test group • 57.1% and 38% of the control group.
Dai et al., 1995 (*182*)	20:18	Randomized controlled trial	Auricular acupuncture at point heart	Auricular acupuncture at point stomach	Marked relief of angina pectoris and other symptoms, with improvement of ECG & haemor-rheological indices was observed in the test group. There was no such effect in the control group.
Cheng, 1995 (*183*)	50:50	Randomized controlled trial	Auricular acupressure	Conventional medication (glyceryl trinitrate, etc.)	A marked effect (no recurrence of angina during the 4–5 weeks of treatment) was observed in: • 74% of the test group • 52% of the control group.

34

4. Summary table of controlled clinical trials

Condition/Study	No.	Design	Test group	Control Group	Results
Ma et al., 1997 (251)	30:24	Randomized controlled trial	Body acupuncture plus routine Western medication (aspirin, nitrates and calcium antagonist)	Routine Western medication (aspirin, nitrates and calcium antagonist)	After 10 days of hospitalization and treatment, improvement in angina pectoris and ST-T, respectively, was observed in : • 85.7% and 69% of the test group • 58.3% and 33.3% of the control group. Levels of serotonin, noradrenaline and dopamine were higher than normal in both groups but were significantly lowered only in test group after the treatment.
Craniocerebral injury, closed Ding et al., 1997 (252)	50:50	Group comparison	Body acupuncture	Routine Western medication (unspecified)	After 15 days of treatment, clinical cure (disappearance of the main clinical symptoms and signs, and basic recovery of functions) was observed in: • 86% of the test group • 56% of the control group.
Deafness, sudden onset Wang et al., 1998 (218)	50:50	Randomized controlled trial	Body acupuncture plus routine Western treatment (dextran, dexamethasone, etc.)	Routine Western medication (dextran, dexamethasone, etc.)	After 2 weeks of treatment, the effect was highly statistically significant in: • 90% of the test group • 70% of the control group.
Defective ejaculation, see Male sexual dysfunction, non-organic					
Shui, 1990 (148)	30:30:40	Randomized controlled trial	Acupuncture	Herbal medication or the Goboes and Liu regimens (treatment included sex instruction, electric massage, hormonal therapy and injection of strychnine and galantamine	After 1 month of treatment, the cure rate was: • 83.3% in the test group • 56.7% in the herbal medication group • 12.5% in the control Goboes and Liu regimen group.
Dental pain Sung et al., 1977 (78) (postoperative)	40	Randomized controlled trial	Acupuncture plus placebo drug	Sham acupuncture plus placebo drug, sham acupuncture plus codeine, or acupuncture plus codeine	Acupuncture plus placebo drug gave significantly greater pain relief than sham acupuncture plus placebo drug or sham acupuncture plus codeine. Acupuncture plus placebo drug was more effective than acupuncture plus codeine in initial 30 min after surgery; less effective 2–3 h after surgery.
Zheng et al., 1990 (79) (after pulp devitalization)	15:11	Randomized controlled trial	Auricular acupressure	No treatment	After 48 h, there was no pain in: • 12/15 (80%) in the test group • 4/11(36%) in the control group.

Acupuncture: review and analysis of controlled clinical trials

Condition/Study	No.	Design	Test group	Control Group	Results
Lao et al., 1995 (77) (after tooth extraction)	11:8	Randomized controlled trial	Acupuncture	Placebo acupuncture	Subjects treated with acupuncture reported a significantly longer period without pain and experienced less intense pain than controls.
Sukandar et al., 1995 (80) (apical periodontitis)	20:20	Randomized controlled trial	Electric acupuncture	Mock electric acupuncture	Analgesic effect lasting 24 h was obtained in: • 65% of the test group • 10% of the control group.
Lao et al, 1999 (73) (after oral surgery)	19:20	Randomized controlled trial	Acupuncture	Placebo acupuncture	Acupuncture was statistically significantly superior to the placebo in preventing postoperative dental pain. Mean pain-free postoperative time and minutes before requesting pain relief medication, respectively, were: • 172.9 min and 242.1 min in the test group • 93.8 min and 166.2 min in the placebo group.
Dependence, alcohol					
Bullock et al., 1987 (210)	27:27	Randomized controlled trial	Acupuncture at specific points	Acupuncture at non-specific points	There was a significant difference between the two groups at the end of the study; patients in the test group expressed less need for alcohol, with fewer drinking episodes.
Bullock et al., 1989 (211)	40:40	Randomized controlled trial	Acupuncture at specific points	Acupuncture at non-specific points	Significant treatment effects persisted at the end of the 6-month follow-up; more control patients expressed a moderate–strong need for alcohol and had more than twice the number of drinking episodes & admissions to detoxification centres.
Dependence, opium, cocaine and heroin					
Margolin et al., 1993 (201) (cocaine)	32 per group	Group comparison (post hoc)	Auricular	Desipramine, amantadine or drug placebo	Abstinence rates during final 2 weeks of 8-week treatment were: • auricular acupuncture 44% • desipramine 26% • amantadine 15% • drug placebo 13%.
Washburn et al., 1993 (202) (heroin)	100	Randomized controlled trial	Acupuncture	Sham acupuncture	Self-reported frequency of heroin use was lower in the test group.
Cai et al., 1998 (200) (heroin, late stage of abstinence)	60:60	Randomized controlled trial	Body acupuncture	Vitamin B_1	Reduction of anorexia, spontaneous sweating and insomnia in the late stage of abstinence was greater in test group, and statistically significant.

4. Summary table of controlled clinical trials

Condition/Study	No.	Design	Test group	Control Group	Results
Bullock et al., 1999 (199) (cocaine)	236	Randomized controlled trial	Auricular acupuncture	Acupuncture at sham ear points or conventional treatment without acupuncture	The data failed to identify significant treatment differences among the various groups.
Dependence, tobacco					
Fang, 1983 (204)	33:28	Randomized controlled trial (patients told they were receiving acupuncture for other purposes)	Auricular acupuncture	Body acupuncture	Under a regime of passive abstinence with no suggestion or motivation, auricular acupuncture was superior to body acupuncture in reducing the tobacco consumption by more than half in: • 70% of the auricular acupuncture group (72% experienced disgust at the taste of tobacco and 15% felt dizzy during smoking) • 11% of the body acupuncture group.
Clavel et al., 1985 (253)	224:205: 222	Randomized group comparison	Acupuncture	Nicotine gum or minimal intervention (cigarette case with lock controlled by a time switch, which could be regulated at will)	Acupuncture and nicotine gum did not reduce the tendency to relapse after one month but were effective in helping smokers to stop smoking during the first month in: • 43/224 in the acupuncture group • 46/205 in the group receiving nicotine gum • 8/222 in the minimal intervention group.
He et al., 1997 (205)	23:23	Randomized controlled trial	Acupuncture at points used to assist smoking cessation	Acupuncture at points assumed to have no effect on smoking cessation	Daily cigarette consumption fell during the treatment in both groups, but the reduction was larger in the test group. Serum concentrations of cotinine and thiocyanate were significantly reduced after the treatment period in the test group but not in the control group.
White et al., 1998 (207)	76	Randomized controlled trial	Electric acupuncture at appropriate points in each ear	Sham procedure (auricular acupuncture over the mastoid bone)	There was no significant difference between the two groups in the mean score for reduction of withdrawal symptoms.
Waite et al., 1998 (206)	78	Randomized controlled trial	Electric acupuncture plus self-retained ear seed (a herbal seed used to apply pressure to the point) at an active site	Auricular acupuncture plus self-retained ear seed at a placebo site	The test acupuncture was significantly more effective in helping volunteers to quit smoking than the control treatment. Cessation of smoking at 6 months in: • 12.5% of the test group • 0% of the control group.
Depression (see also Depression after stroke)					
Luo et al., 1985 (191)	27:20	Randomized controlled trial	Electric acupuncture	Medication (amitriptyline)	There was a similar improvement in the two groups but far fewer side-effects in the test group.

37

Condition/Study	No.	Design	Test group	Control Group	Results
Luo et al., 1988 (192)	133:108	Multicentre, randomized controlled trial	Electric acupuncture	Medication (amitriptyline)	There was a similar improvement in the two groups but a greater effect on anxiety and fewer side-effects in the test group.
Yang et al., 1994 (193)	20:20	Randomized controlled trial	Acupuncture	Medication (amitriptyline)	There was a similar improvement in the two groups after 6 weeks.
Luo et al., 1998 (254)	29	Randomized controlled trial	Electric acupuncture plus placebo	Electric acupuncture plus amitriptyline	The therapeutic efficacy was similar in the two groups for depressive disorders. The therapeutic effect for anxiety somatization and cognitive process disturbance was greater and there were fewer side-effects in the test group.
Depression after stroke					
Li et al., 1994 (190)	34:34: 33	Randomized controlled trial	"Antidepressive" acupuncture (different selection of points)	Medication (doxepin) plus traditional acupuncture or traditional acupuncture alone	There was a similar improvement in the anti-depressive acupuncture and medication plus traditional acupuncture groups; improvement was superior to that in traditional acupuncture group.
Hou et al., 1996 (189)	30:30	Randomized controlled trial with independent assessment	Electric acupuncture at *bǎihuì* (GV20) and *yìntáng* (EX-HN3)	Traditional manual acupuncture	The results were better in the test group; the difference was significant as assessed by the Hamilton and other scoring methods.
Depressive neurosis					
Zhang, 1996 (194)	31 per group	Randomized controlled trial	Laser acupuncture	Conventional antidepressant (doxepin, amitriptyline or aprazolam)	The therapeutic effect was similar in the two groups, somewhat better in the test group for cognitive disturbance. Side-effects occurred in all cases in control group but in none in test group.
Diabetes mellitus, non-insulin-dependent					
Latief, 1987 (241)	20:20	Randomized controlled trial	Acupuncture at *sānyīnjiāo* (SP6)	Acupuncture at 1 Chinese inch (*cun*) superiolateral to SP6	There was a reduction in fasting blood sugar of: • 19.2% in the test group • 4.9% in the control group.
Kang et al., 1995 (240)	12:15: 13:10	Randomized controlled trial	Untimed acupuncture or acupuncture at insulin secretion climax (ISCA) or acupuncture at insulin secretion valley (ICSV)	Conventional Western medication (tolbutamide)	Improvement in fasting blood glucose, 2-h glucose, postprandial blood glucose, 24-h urine glucose, and glucosylated haemoglobin was: • marked in the ISCA group • superior in the ISCA group to that in the untimed acupuncture and ISVA groups • similar in the ISCA group to that of the tolbutamide group.

4. Summary table of controlled clinical trials

Condition/Study	No.	Design	Test group	Control Group	Results
Diarrhoea, see Diarrhoea in infants and children; Dysentery, acute bacillary; Irritable colon syndrome					
Diarrhoea in infants and young children					
Li et al., 1997 (213)	380:450	Group comparison	Acupuncture at *zúsānlǐ* (ST36) and *chángqiáng* (GV1)	Medication (gentamicin or haloperidol)	Cure in 1 day was obtained in: • 82.3% of the test group (the remainder were cured within 3 days) • 41.3% of the control group.
Yang, 1998 (214)	100:70	Group comparison	Body acupuncture and moxibustion	Medication (antibiotics and vitamins)	Cure was obtained in: • 98% of test group within 3.43 ± 0.32 days • 80% of control group within 4.41 ± 0.43 days.
Dysentery, acute bacillary					
Qiu et al., 1986 (9)	596:281	Group comparison	Acupuncture	Medication (furazolidone)	Acupuncture relieved symptoms earlier than furazolidone. Stool culture became negative in: • 92.4% of the test group • 98.2% of the control group.
Li, 1990 (8)	276:269	Group comparison	Acupuncture	Medication (syntomycin, furazolidone)	Stool culture became negative in all patients after 7 days, but within 7 days in: • 87.7% of the test group; recurrence rate in 1 year, 2.4% • 74.2% of the control group; recurrence rate in 1 year, 2.5%.
Yu et al., 1992 (10)	162:164	Randomized controlled trial	Acupuncture	Medication (furazolidone)	Both treatments relieved symptoms and signs, with no side-effects. Stool culture became negative in: • 128 (79%) in the test group by 5.1 days; recurrence at 9-month follow-up in 4 cases • 143 (87.2%) in the control group by 3.2 days; recurrence at 9-month follow-up in 5 cases.
Dysmenorrhoea, primary					
Helms, 1987 (153)	11:11:11:10	Randomized controlled trial, comparing four groups	Acupuncture	Placebo acupuncture, no acupuncture but conventional treatment, no acupuncture but conventional treatment and control visits to physician	Improvement was observed in: • 10/11(90.9%) in the real acupuncture group • 4/11 (36.4%) in the placebo acupuncture group • 2/11 (18.2%) in the conventional treatment control group • 1/10 (10%) in the conventional treatment plus visits control group.

Acupuncture: review and analysis of controlled clinical trials

Condition/Study	No.	Design	Test group	Control Group	Results
Shi et al., 1994 (154)	120:44	Randomized controlled trial	Acupuncture at sānyīnjiāo (SP6)	Medication (a paracetamol–propyphenazone–caffeine combination)	A better and quicker analgesic effect was observed in the test group.
Dysphagia in pseudobulbar paralysis					
Liu et al., 1998 (255)	30:30	Randomized controlled trial	Body acupuncture	Logemann functional training of lingual muscles	Cure rates after 15 days were: • 26 in the test group (average 8.7 days) • 6 in the control group.
Earache, unexplained					
Mekhamer A et al. 1987 (222)	96	Randomized controlled trial	Acupuncture	Mock TENS	The response was significantly better following acupuncture than placebo for both 33% and 50% pain-relief criteria.
Encephalitis, see Viral encephalitis in children					
Epidemic haemorrhagic fever					
Song et al., 1992 (86)	38:32	Randomized controlled trial	Moxibustion	Western medication. (steroid, supportive treatment)	Moxibustion shortened the period of oliguria and accelerated the fall in urine protein and reduction in kidney swelling (ultrasound).
Epigastralgia, acute (in peptic ulcer, acute and chronic gastritis, and gastrospasm)					
Xu et al., 1991 (128)	42:31	Randomized controlled trial	Acupuncture at liángqiū (ST34) and wèishū (BL21)	Conventional medication. (anisodamine)	The treatment was effective in: • 97.6% of the test group • 83.9% of the control group.
Yu, 1997 (129)	160:40	Randomized controlled trial	Acupuncture (manual) at zúsānlǐ (ST36)	Medication (morphine plus atropine)	A marked effect was observed in: • 81% of the test group • 80% of the control group.
Epistaxis, simple (without generalized or local disease)					
Lang et al., 1995 (223)	92:42	Randomized controlled trial	Auricular acupuncture with thumb-tack needle	Western medication (carbazochrome salicylate plus vitamin C)	Cure (no recurrence at 3-month follow-up) was observed in: • 84.8% of the test group • 28.6% of the control group.
Eye pain due to subconjunctival injection					
Shen, 1996 (14)	24:15	Randomized controlled trial	Acupuncture at bìnào (LI14)	No treatment	Pain mostly disappeared in 0.5–1 min in 22/24 of the test group but persisted for 30–60 min in all of the control patients.
Facial pain (including craniomandibular disorders) (see also Temporomandibular joint dysfunction)					
Hansen et al., 1983 (29)	16	Randomized crossover trial	Acupuncture	Sham acupuncture	Pain levels were more significantly reduced following acupuncture than following sham acupuncture.

40

4. Summary table of controlled clinical trials

Condition/Study	No.	Design	Test group	Control Group	Results
Johansson et al., 1991 (30)	15 per group	Randomized controlled trial	Acupuncture	Occlusal splint or no treatment	Acupuncture was as effective as occlusal splint. At follow-up, subjective dysfunction scores and visual analogue scale assessments were significantly lower in the test group.
List, 1992 (31)	110	Randomized controlled trial	Acupuncture.	Occlusal splint or no treatment	Symptoms were reduced by acupuncture and occlusal-splint therapy. The control group remained essentially unchanged. Acupuncture gave better short-term subjective results than occlusal splint.
Cai, 1996 (28)	32:36	Randomized controlled trial	Acupuncture with retention of needles for 1–1.5 h	Acupuncture with retention of needles for 0.5 h	Marked effect (with effective rate after course of treatment of 14 sessions): • 59.3% of test group after 5 sessions of treatment; overall effective rate, 93.7% • 25% of the control group after 11 sessions on average; overall effective rate, 77.8%.
Facial spasm					
Liu, 1996 (107)	33:33	Randomized controlled trial	Wrist–ankle acupuncture	Body acupuncture	Elimination of involuntary twitching with no recurrence at 6-month follow-up in: • 69.7% of the test group • 39.4 % of the control group.
Female urethral syndrome					
Zheng et al., 1997 (151)	103:50	Randomized controlled trial	Body acupuncture and moxibustion.	Medication (Urgenin: herbal extract containing *Serenoa serrulata*, effective for irritable bladder; used because antibiotics had proved ineffective in all patients)	Effective rates after 1–2 months of treatment were: • 88.3% in the test group • 28% in the control group.
Wang et al., 1998 (150) (from same institute as study above)	56:37	Randomized controlled trial	Body acupuncture and moxibustion	Medication. (Urgenin; used because antibiotics had proved ineffective)	Effective rates after 1–2 months of treatment were: • 87.5% in the test group (urodynamic study also showed the beneficial effect of acupuncture) • 29.7% in the control group.

Acupuncture: review and analysis of controlled clinical trials

Condition/Study	No.	Design	Test group	Control Group	Results
Fever, see Convulsions in infants and young children due to high fever; Tonsillitis, acute					
Fibromyalgia					
Deluze et al.,1992 (*40*)	36:34	Randomized controlled trial with independent assessment	Acupuncture	Sham acupuncture	There was a significant difference between the two groups with improvement in: • 7 of the 8 parameters in the test group • none of the parameters in the control group.
Gastrointestinal spasm					
Shi et al., 1995 (*130*)	100:100	Randomized controlled trial	Acupuncture	Atropine	Total relief of pain in 30 min was observed in: • 98 in the test group • 71 in the control group.
Gastrokinetic disturbance					
Zhang et al., 1996 (*131*)	104:41	Randomized controlled trial	Acupuncture	Conventional medication (domperidone)	Effective rates (no significant difference between the two groups) were: • 95.2% in the test group • 90.2% in the control group.
Gouty arthritis					
Li et al., 1993 (*60*)	23:19	Randomized controlled trial	Blood-pricking acupuncture	Conventional medication (allopurinol)	The test group showed more marked improvement than the control group. Reduction in blood and urine uric acid was similar in the two groups.
Pan, 1997 (*61*)	39:20	Randomized controlled trial	Plum-blossom needling plus cupping	Medication (allopurinol)	After 6 weeks of treatment, marked improvement was observed in: • 100% of the test group • 65% of the control group.
Haemorrhagic fever, see Epidemic haemorrhagic fever					
Hay fever, see Allergic rhinitis (including hay fever)					
Headache					
Ahonen et al., 1983 (*17*) (myogenic)	12:10	Group comparison	Acupuncture	Physiotherapy	Significant changes in pain and electromyogram in both groups, with 4 sessions of acupuncture equivalent to 8 sessions of physiotherapy.
Loh et al., 1984 (*23*) (migraine and tension)	48	Crossover (incomplete)	Acupuncture	Standard drug therapy (mainly propranolol)	Benefit was observed in: • 59% of the test group; 39% with marked improvement • 25% of the control group; 11% with marked improvement.

4. Summary table of controlled clinical trials

Condition/Study	No.	Design	Test group	Control Group	Results
Dowson et al., 1985 (20) (migraine)	25:23	Randomized controlled trial	Acupuncture	Mock TENS	33% severity improvement was observed in: • 56% (14/25) of the acupuncture group • 30% (7/23) of the control group. Headache frequency was reduced in: • 44% (11/25) of the acupuncture group • 57% (13/23) of the control group.
Doerr-Proske et al., 1985 (19) (migraine)	10 per group	Randomized controlled trial	Acupuncture	Psychological biobehavioural treatment or no treatment (on waiting list)	Over 3 months of treatment, there was a significant reduction of headache frequency and intensity in the acupuncture and psychological biobehavioural groups. There was almost no change in those on the waiting list.
Vincent, 1989 (25) (migraine)	15:15	Randomized controlled trial	Acupuncture	Sham acupuncture	There was a significant difference between two groups: the test group experienced sustained improvement over 1 year after only 6 treatments in a 6-week period.
Tavola et al., 1992 (24) (tension)	15:15	Randomized controlled trial	Acupuncture	Sham acupuncture	The mean decreases in headache episodes, headache index and analgesic intake, respectively were: • 44.3%, 58.3% and 57.7% in the test group • 21.4%, 27.8% and 21.7% in the control group.
Kubiena et al., 1992 (21) (migraine)	15:15	Randomized controlled trial	Acupuncture	Placebo acupuncture	The test group showed better results than the control group (reduction in frequency of attacks, intensity of pain and amount of medication taken).
Xu et al., 1993 (27) (migraine)	50:50	Randomized group comparison	Manual acupuncture	Electric acupuncture	There was an Immediate analgesic effect in: • 80% of the test group • 48% of the control group.
Weinschütz et al., 1994 (26) (migraine)	20:20	Controlled trial, comparable pretreatment conditions	Acupuncture at classical points	Acupuncture at points 1–2 cm from those used in test group	Acupuncture at classical points yielded a significant therapeutic effect superior to the control acupuncture.
Chen et al., 1997 (18) (migraine)	45:30	Group comparison	Penetrating acupuncture	Nimodipine	After 20 days of treatment, headache disappeared with no recurrence after 6 months of follow-up in: • 30/45 in the test group • 16/30 in the control group.

Acupuncture: review and analysis of controlled clinical trials

Condition/Study	No.	Design	Test group	Control Group	Results
Liu et al., 1997 (22) (migraine)	30:34	Randomized controlled trial	Scalp acupuncture	Flunarizine	Headache was relieved after 1 week treatment in: • 73.3% of the test group • 38.2% of the control group.
Heart disease, see Coronary heart disease (angina pectoris); Pulmonary heart disease, chronic					
Hepatitis B virus carrier Wang et al., 1991 (85)	70:42	Group comparison	Acupuncture plus moxibustion	Herbal medication (Herba Cymbopogonis)	After 3 months of treatment, carrier status became negative in: • 30% of the test group • 2.4% of the control group. Antibodies to hepatitis B e core antigen were produced in: • 50% of the test group • 6.25% of the control group.
Heroin dependence, see Dependence, opium, cocaine, heroin					
Herpes zoster (human (alpha) herpesvirus 3) (see also Neuralgia, post-herpetic) Chen et al., 1994 (225)	33:32	Randomized controlled trial	Laser acupuncture	Polyinosinic acid	Disappearance of pain and formation of scabs, respectively, occurred after: • 1.48 and 5.76 days of laser acupuncture • 10.5 and 10.4 days of medication.
Hyperlipaemia Wang, 1998 (239)	40:25	Group comparison	Acupoint injection plus oral administration of simvastatin	Oral administration of simvastatin	Significant improvement after 30 days of treatment in: • 36/40 (90%) in the test group • 11/25 (44%) in the control group.
Hypertension, essential Iurenev et al., 1988 (173)	25:38	Group comparison	Acupuncture	Conventional medication (rescinnamine)	The therapeutic efficacy was similar in the two groups.
Zhou et al., 1990 (176)	135:68:71	Group comparison	Auricular acupressure	Medication (nifedipine plus propranolol) or placebo drug	There was a similar improvement with acupressure and medication. Both were superior to placebo.
Yu et al, 1991 (175)	280:51	Group comparison	Auricular acupressure	Conventional medication (reserpine)	There was a similar improvement in the two groups. There were no side-effects in the test group.

4. Summary table of controlled clinical trials

Condition/Study	No.	Design	Test group	Control Group	Results
Wu et al., 1997 (*174*)	82:118	Group comparison	Scalp acupuncture	Conventional medication (nifedipine)	The effects were similar, with no statistically significant difference, in the two groups: • marked response in 47.6%, partial response in 50% of the test group • marked response in 57.6%, partial response in 40.7% of the control group.
Dan, 1998 (*172*)	26:26	Randomized controlled trial	Acupuncture	Conventional medication (nifedipine)	Monitoring of ambulatory blood pressure showed a similar reduction in 24-h systolic and diastolic blood pressure in the two groups. The reduction in myocardial oxygen consumption index was greater in the test group.
Hypo-ovarianism Ma et al., 1997 (*256*)	30:30	Randomized controlled trial	Body acupuncture (manual) plus cupping	Medication (diethylstilbestrol)	Marked improvement was observed in: • 43/56 (76.8%) in the test group (hormonal assay showed a further long-term effect after treatment) • 26/55 (47.3%) in the diethylstilbestrol group.
Hypophrenia Tian et al., 1996 (*254*)	100:25	Randomized controlled trial	Body plus ear acupuncture plus application of herbal extract to acupoints	No treatment	Intelligence quotient increased: • from 53.97 to 65.07 (11.10 $\pm$ 2.96) in the test group • from 53.87 to 55.12 in the control group. Social adaptability behaviour increased: • from 7.51 to 8.89 (1.38 $\pm$ 0.31) in test group • from 7.57 to 7.82 in the control group.
Hypotension, primary Guo, 1992 (*170*)	50:50	Randomized controlled trial	Auricular acupressure	Herbal tonics	After 10 days of treatment, blood pressure was restored to normal in: • 45 in the study group (no improvement in 1) • 15 in the control group (no improvement in 25).
Yu et al., 1998 (*171*)	180:60	Randomized controlled trial	Acupuncture at *bǎihuì* (GV20) plus herbal medication (*Bu Zhong Yi Qi Tang*, a formula that is routinely used in herbal medicine for the treatment of hypotension)	Herbal medication (*Bu Zhong Yi Qi Tang*)	A therapeutic effect was observed after 0.5–1 month of treatment in: • 172/180 (95.5%) in the test group • 46/60 (76.7%) in the control group.

Acupuncture: review and analysis of controlled clinical trials

Condition/Study	No.	Design	Test group	Control Group	Results
Induction of labour					
Yu et al., 1981 (*161*)	10:10:8	Randomized group comparison	Acupuncture at distant points or local points	Acupuncture at distant plus local points	Acupuncture at distant points was superior to that at local points in strengthening uterine contractions for induction of labour. Combined use of distant & local points was best technique.
Lin et al., 1992 (*159*)	62:48	Randomized controlled trial	Acupuncture at *hégǔ* (LI4) and *sānyīnjiāo* (SP6)	Oxytocin intravenous drip	Similar results were obtained in the two groups, but uterine contractions were less frequent and uterine motility was less marked in the test group.
Ma et al., 1995 (*160*)	31:29: 15:26	Randomized controlled trial	(1) Ear acupuncture at *shénmén*, (2) Body acupuncture at *sānyīnjiāo* (SP6) or (3) Body acupuncture at *yánglíngquán* (GB34)	(4) No treatment	The duration of labour in the four groups was: • (1) 4.47 ± 0.76 h • (2) 6.80 ± 1.04 h • (3) 9.79 ± 2.45 h • (4) 10.20 ± 2.04 h.
Infertility, see Defective ejaculation; Hypo-ovarianism; Infertility due to inflammatory obstruction of fallopian tube; Male sexual dysfunction, non-organic					
Infertility due to inflammatory obstruction of fallopian tube					
Ji et al., 1996 (*158*)	64:36:30	Randomized controlled trial	Manual acupuncture plus electric acupuncture plus moxibustion	Herbal medication or conventional Western medication (intrauterine injection of gentamicin, chymotrypsin and dexamethasone)	Results showed that the fallopian tube obstruction was totally removed in: • 81.3% of the test group; in a 2-year follow-up, the pregnancy rate was 75% • 55.6% and 56.7% of the control groups, respectively; in a 2-years follow-up, the pregnancy rates were 52.7% and 46.7%.
Insomnia					
Zhang, 1993 (*110*)	60 per group	Group comparison	Auricular acupressure	Medication (diazepam plus chlorohydrate)	After 1 month of treatment, sleep was restored to normal or markedly improved in: • 59/60 in the test group • 20/60 in the control group.
Luo et al., 1993 (*109*)	60 per group	Randomized controlled trial	Auricular acupressure	Medication (phenobarbital, methaqualone or meprobamate)	After the course of treatment, sleep improved in: • 96.7% of the test group • 35.0% of the control group.
Irritable bladder, see Female urethral syndrome					
Irritable colon syndrome					
Wu et al., 1996 (*133*)	41:40	Randomized controlled trial	Moxibustion	Western medication	After 2.5–3 months of treatment, a therapeutic effect was observed in: • 92.7% of test group (improvement in 53.7%) • 62.5% of control group (improvement in 37.5%).

4. Summary table of controlled clinical trials

Condition/Study	No.	Design	Test group	Control Group	Results
Knee pain					
Maruno, 1976 (*56*) (arthrosis)	26:26	Randomized controlled trial	Electric acupuncture	Manual acupuncture	Good results (complete alleviation of pain) were observed in: • 17/26 in the test group (average no. of treatments required, 6) • 11/26 in the control group (average no. of treatments required, 10).
Christensen et al., 1992 (*54*) (osteoarthritis)	14:15	Randomized controlled trial, independent assessment	Acupuncture	No treatment (waiting for surgery)	Reduction in pain, analgesic consumption and objective measurements were significantly greater in the test group.
Berman et al., 1999 (*58*) (osteoarthritis)	73	Randomized controlled trial	Acupuncture	Standard care (weight loss, physical and occupational therapy, medication)	Improvement according to the Western Ontario and McMaster Universities Osteoarthritis Index and Lequesne indices was superior in test group.
Labour, see Induction of labour; Labour pain					
Labour pain					
Zhang et al., 1995 (*82*)	150:150	Randomized controlled trial with independent assessment	Body plus ear acupuncture	No treatment	Acupuncture yielded a good analgesic effect and expedited the opening of the uterine ostium.
Lactation deficiency					
Chandra et al., 1995 (*169*)	15:15	Randomized controlled trial	Electric acupuncture	No acupuncture	Lactation increased by: • 92% in the test group • 30.9% in the control group. The difference was statistically significant.
Leukopenia					
Chen et al., 1991 (*141*) (chemotherapy-induced)	121:117:34	Randomized controlled trial	Acupuncture or moxibustion	Medication (batilol plus cysteine phenylacetate)	Effective rates after 9 days of treatment were: • 88.4% in the acupuncture group • 91.5% in the moxibustion group • 38.2% in the medication group.
Chen et al., 1990 (*140*) (chemotherapy-induced)	57:34	Randomized controlled trial	Moxibustion	Medication (batilol plus cysteine-phenylacetate)	Effective rates after 9 days of treatment were: • 89.5% in the test group • 38.2% in the control group.
Yin et al., 1990 (*143*) (benzene-induced)	30:27	Randomized controlled trial	Acupuncture	Medication (cysteine-phenylacetate)	Effective rates after 6 weeks of treatment were: • 83.3% in the test group • 53.4% in the control group.

Acupuncture: review and analysis of controlled clinical trials

Condition/Study	No.	Design	Test group	Control Group	Results
Yin et al., 1992 (*144*) (benzene-induced)	30:25	Randomized controlled trial	Acupuncture	Medication (rubidate)	Acupuncture was superior to rubidate in improving symptoms and increasing leukocyte count; effective rates were: • 91% in the test group • 68% in the control group.
Wang, 1997 (*142*) (chemotherapy-induced)	49:34	Randomized controlled trial	Moxibustion	Medication (batilol plus cysteine-phenylacetate)	Effective rates were: • 82% in the test group • 50% in the control group.
Low back pain (see also Sciatica; Spine pain, acute)					
Gunn et al., 1980 (*46*)	29:27	Randomized controlled trial	Acupuncture	Standard therapy (physical therapy, remedial exercises, etc.)	Return to original or equivalent work or to lighter work, respectively, was possible in: • 18/29 and 10/29 in the test group • 4/27 and 14/27 in the control group.
Coan et al., 1980 (*45*)	25:25	Randomized controlled trial	Acupuncture and electric acupuncture	No treatment (waiting list)	Improvement was observed in: • 19/25 in the test group • 5/25 in the control group.
Mendelson et al., 1983 (*49*)	95	Randomized single-blind crossover with independent assessment	Acupuncture	Lidocaine injection plus sham acupuncture	Improvement was observed in: • 26 in the test group • 22 in the control group.
MacDonald et al., 1983 (*48*)	8:9	Randomized controlled trial	Acupuncture and electric acupuncture	Mock TENS	Combined average reduction (pain score, activity pain, physical signs) was: • 71.4% in the acupuncture group • 21.4% in the control group.
Lehmann et al., 1986 (*47*)	17:18:18	Randomized controlled trial	Electric acupuncture	TENS or mock TENS	There was a significantly greater gain in various measures in the test group during a 3-week in-patient treatment period and at 6-month follow-up.
Male sexual dysfunction, non-organic (see also Defective ejaculation)					
Aydin et al., 1997 (*147*)	15:16:29	Randomized controlled trial	Acupuncture	Hypnosis or placebo	Success rates were: • 60% in the acupuncture group • 75% in the group treated with hypnotic suggestion • 43–47% in the placebo group.

4. Summary table of controlled clinical trials

Condition/Study	No.	Design	Test group	Control Group	Results
Malposition of fetus, correction of					
Qin et al., 1989[(167)	100:40	Group comparison	Auricular acupressure	Knee-chest position	Success rates were: • 92.9% in the test group • 67.5% in the control group.
Li et al., 1990 (165)	27:27:20	Group comparison	Moxibustion at zúlínqì (GB41)	Moxibustion at zhìyīn (BL67) (not traditionally used for fetal transposition) or at a non-classical point (located 3 cm below the head of the fibula)	After 1 week of treatment, successful transposition occurred in: • 51.9% of the test group • 22.2% and 15%, respectively, in the control groups.
Li et al., 1996 (166)	48:31	Group comparison	Electric acupuncture at zhìyīn (BL67)	No treatment	Efficacy was markedly superior in the test group.
Cardini et al., 1998 (164)	130:130	Randomized controlled trial	Moxibustion at zhìyīn (BL67)	Routine care but no intervention for breech presentation	Among primigravidas with breech presentation during the 33rd week of gestation, moxibustion for 1–2 weeks increased fetal activity during the treatment period and resulted in cephalic presentation after treatment period & at delivery.
Ménière disease					
Zhang et al., 1983 (219)	33:32	Randomized controlled trial with partial crossover	Acupuncture	Conventional Western medication (betahistine, nicotinic acid, vitamin B_6, cinnarizine)	After 15 days of treatment, the syndrome was relieved in: • 25 in the test group (ameliorated in 1), with relief usually occurring immediately after treatment • 16 in the control group (ameliorated in 2). Of the 7 unaffected acupuncture patients, 5 returned to receive medication; all remained unimproved. Of the 14 unaffected control patients, 6 returned to receive acupuncture; 2 were cured and 1 improved. Effective rates were: • 74.4% in 39 courses of acupuncture treatment • 48.6% in 37 courses of medication.
Migraine, see Headache					
Morning sickness (see also Nausea and vomiting)					
Dundee et al., 1988 (162)	119:112: 119	Randomized controlled trial	Acupressure at nèiguān (PC6) or sham acupressure (a point near right elbow)	No treatment	Troublesome sickness was significantly less in the acupressure (23/119) and sham acupressure (41/112) groups than in the control group (67/119).

49

Acupuncture: review and analysis of controlled clinical trials

Condition/Study	No.	Design	Test group	Control Group	Results
De Aloysio et al., 1992 (258)	66	Randomized controlled trial	Acupressure at nèiguān (PC6)	Sham acupressure	Effective rates were: • 60% in the test group • 30% in the control group.
Bayreuther et al., 1994 (259)	23	Randomized single-blind crossover with independent assessment	Acupressure at nèiguān (PC6)	Sham acupressure	Effective rates were: • 69% in the test group • 31% in the control group.
Fan, 1995 (163)	151:151	Randomized group comparison	Moxibustion	Herbal medication	Cure rates after 1 week of treatment were: • 96.7% in the test group • 58.9% in the control group.
Nausea and vomiting (see also Adverse reactions to radiotherapy and/or chemotherapy; Morning sickness)					
Dundee et al., 1986 (260) (peri- and postoperative)	25 per group	Group comparison	(1) Acupuncture plus meptazinol, (2) Acupuncture plus nalbuphine	(3) Meptazinol (4) Sham acupuncture plus nalbuphine (5) Nalbuphine	Vomiting in group (1) was half that in group (3). There was a significantly lower incidence of emetic episodes in the acupuncture groups (1) and (2) than in the control groups (3), (4) and (5). There were no differences between the control groups (3), (4) and (5).
Dundee et al., 1987 (233) (cisplatin-associated)	10	Randomized crossover trial	Electric acupuncture at nèiguān (PC6)	Electric acupuncture at "dummy" point	Sickness was significantly lower in the test group.
Ghaly et al., 1987 261) (postoperative)	31:31	Group comparison	Acupuncture plus electric acupuncture	Medication (cyclizine)	Acupuncture and electric acupuncture were as effective as medication.
Weightman et al., 1987 (262) (postoperative)	46	Double-blind randomized controlled trial	Acupuncture at nèiguān (PC6)	No acupuncture	Acupuncture performed during surgery under anaesthesia did not lead to a significant reduction in nausea or vomiting after surgery.
Dundee et al., 1989 (263) (chemotherapy-related)	20	Group comparison	Acupuncture at nèiguān (PC6)	Sham acupuncture	Effective rates were: • 90% in the test group • 10% in the control group.
Barsoum et al., 1990 (264) (postoperative)	162	Randomized controlled trial	Acupressure at nèiguān (PC6) by using bands (with pressure button)	Placebo bands (without pressure button) or injection of prochlorperazine	The severity of nausea was significantly reduced in the test group compared with the two control groups.

4. Summary table of controlled clinical trials

Condition/Study	No.	Design	Test group	Control Group	Results
Ho et al., 1990 (265) (postoperative)	25 per group	Group comparison	Electric acupuncture	Medication (intravenous prochlorperazine 5 mg) or TENS or no treatment	Emesis episodes were observed in: • 3/25 in the electric acupuncture group • 3/25 in the medication group • 9/25 in the TENS group • 11/25 in the untreated group.
Ho et al., 1996 (266) (postoperative)	60	Randomized double-blind controlled trial	Acupressure bands (with pressure button)	Placebo bands (without pressure button)	Incidence of nausea and of vomiting, respectively was: • 3% and 0% in the test group • 43% and 27% in the control group.
Andrzejowski et al., 1996 (267) (postoperative)	36	Randomized controlled trial	Acupuncture with semipermanent needles	Placebo with needles inserted into sham points	Semipermanent acupuncture did not reduce the overall incidence of nausea and vomiting after abdominal hysterectomy but did reduce the severity of nausea in the second 24-h period and had a greater effect on patients who had nausea & vomiting after a previous anaesthetic.
McConaghy et al., 1996 (268) (postoperative)	30:50	Randomized controlled trial	Acupuncture at nèiguān (PC6)	Acupuncture at sham points	Patients were treated with acupuncture with manual stimulation for 4 min after developing post-operative nausea & vomiting lasting more than 10 min: • 53% of patients in the test group did not require further antiemetic treatment • all patients in the control group required further antiemetic treatment.
Schwager et al., 1996 (269) (postoperative)	84	Randomized controlled trial	Acupuncture	Placebo (no needle stimulation)	There was no statistically significant difference in total postoperative vomiting between the two groups.
Liu et al., 1997 (270) (cisplatin-associated)	184: 161:25: 25:23: 22:70	Randomized group comparison	Magnetic plate at nèiguān (PC6): (1) 120 mT, (2) 60 mT or (3) 2000 mT	(4) 120 mT magnetic plate at zúsānlǐ (ST36), (5) iron plate at nèiguān (PC6), (6) steel bead at nèiguān (PC6) or (7) medication (unspecified)	Total effective rates were significantly higher in the first two test groups): • (1) 92.4% • (2) 89.4% • other group rates ranged from 47.2% (7) to 0%.

Acupuncture: review and analysis of controlled clinical trials

Condition/Study	No.	Design	Test group	Control Group	Results
Al-Sadi et al., 1997 (271) (postoperative)	81	Randomized controlled trial	Acupuncture	Placebo (no needle stimulation)	The use of acupuncture reduced the incidence of postoperative nausea or vomiting in hospital from 65% to 35% (for day cases) and from 69% to 31% (after discharge).
Stein et al., 1997 (272) (postoperative)	75	Randomized double-blind controlled trial	Acupressure bands plus intravenous saline	Placebo bands plus intravenous metoclopramide or placebo bands plus intravenous saline	Patients who received either acupressure or placebo bands plus metoclopramide prior to initiation of spinal anaesthesia for caesarean section experienced much less nausea than patients in the placebo band plus saline group.
Schlager et al., 1998 (273) (postoperative)	40:20	Randomized double-blind controlled trial	Laser stimulation of nèiguān (PC6)	Placebo laser	The incidence of vomiting after strabismus surgery was significantly different for • 25% in the test group • 85% in the control group.
Chu et al., 1998 (274) (postoperative)	34:31	Randomized controlled trial assessed by evaluator blind to treatment	Acupressure using non-invasive vital point needleless acuplaster (Koa, Japan)	Placebo acupressure	The overall incidence of vomiting in a 24-h period after strabismus surgery was: • 29.4% in the test group • 64.5% in the control group.
Alkaissi et al., 1999 (275) (postoperative)	20:20:20	Randomized controlled trial	Acupressure with wrist band	Placebo with or without wrist band	Nausea decreased after 24 h in all groups but vomiting and need of relief antiemetic was reduced only in the test group.
Shenkman et al., 1999 (276) (postoperative)	100	Randomized controlled trial	Acupuncture plus acupressure	Acupuncture at sham points	Perioperative acupressure and acupuncture did not diminish emesis in children following tonsillectomy.
Neck pain					
Coan et al., 1982 (35)	15:15	Randomized controlled trial	Acupuncture plus electric acupuncture	No treatment (waiting list)	Mean pain scores were reduced by: • 40% in the test group; improvement in 12/15 • 2% in the control group; improvement in 2/15.
Loy, 1983 (36)	26:27	Randomized controlled trial	Electric acupuncture	Physiotherapy	Improvement was observed in: • 67.4% of the test group at 3 weeks, 87.2% at 6 weeks • 51.3% of the control group at 3 weeks, 53.9% at 6 weeks.

4. Summary table of controlled clinical trials

Condition/Study	No.	Design	Test group	Control Group	Results
Petrie et al., 1986 (37)	13:12	Randomized controlled trial	Acupuncture	Mock TENS	At 1-month follow-up, daily pill count and disability scores, respectively: • decreased by 23.5% and 24.6% in the test group • increased by 8.4% and 8.4% in control group.
David et al., 1998 (34)	35:35	Randomized controlled trial	Acupuncture	Physiotherapy	Both groups improved in respect of pain and range of movement of neck. Acupuncture was slightly more effective in patients who had higher baseline pain scores.
Birch et al., 1998 (33)	46	Randomized controlled trial	Acupuncture at specific sites relevant for neck pain or acupuncture at specific sites not relevant for neck pain	Nonsteroid anti-inflammatory medication	Relevant acupuncture contributed to modest pain reduction in persons with myofascial neck pain. The relevant acupuncture group had significantly greater pre- and post-treatment differences in pain than the non-relevant acupuncture and medication groups.
Neuralgia, post-herpetic					
Lewith et al., 1983 (103)	30:32	Randomized controlled trial	Auricular plus body acupuncture	Placebo (mock TENS)	There were no differences in the pain recorded in the two groups during or after treatment. There was a significant improvement in pain at the end of treatment in 7 patients of the placebo group and 7 patients of the acupuncture group.
Sukandar et al., 1995 (104)	7:7	Randomized controlled trial	Acupuncture at *jiájĭ* (EX-B2) on affected side plus amitriptyline–trifluoperazine combo (amitriptyline 5 mg + trifluoperazine 0.5 mg per tablet), one tablet twice a day	Acupuncture at *jiájĭ* (EX-B2) on contralateral side plus an amitriptyline–trifluoperazine combination	There was a significant difference in analgesia between the test and control groups. Analgesia was excellent in: • all patients in the test group after 6 sessions • none of the patients in the control group.
Neurodermatitis					
Huang et al., 1998 (227)	60:60	Randomized controlled trial	Acupuncture with seven-star needles	Conventional local treatment	Cure rates were: • 100% in the test group • 16.7% in the control group.
Neuropathic bladder in spinal cord injury					
Cheng et al., 1998 (277)	40:40	Controlled trial	Electric acupuncture	Conventional bladder-training programme	Times taken to achieve balanced voiding were: • 57.1 ± 22.6 days in the test group • 85.2 ± 27.4 days in the control group. The difference was statistically significant.

Condition/Study	No.	Design	Test group	Control Group	Results
Obesity (see also Simple obesity in children)					
Richards et al., 1998 (238)	60	Randomized controlled trial	Auricular acupuncture	Sham acupuncture	Suppression of appetite was noticed in: • 95% of the test group • 0% of the control group.
Opium dependence, see Dependence, opium, cocaine, heroin					
Osteoarthritis					
Junnila, 1982 (55)	16:16	Group comparison (sequential)	Acupuncture	Medication (piroxicam)	Pain was relieved by: • 61% 1 month after a series of acupuncture treatments; no side-effects • 32% after 4 months of piroxicam therapy; itching of the skin, intestinal bleeding, or tiredness occurred in 19%.
Pain, see Abdominal pain in acute gastroenteritis; Biliary colic; Cancer pain; Dental pain; Dysmenorrhoea, primary; Earache; Epigastralgia, acute; Eye pain due to subconjunctival injection; Facial pain (including craniomandibular disorders); Gastrointestinal spasm; Headache; Knee pain; Labour pain; Low back pain; Neck pain; Neuralgia, post-herpetic; Osteoarthritis; Pain due to endoscopic examination; Periarthritis of shoulder; Plantar pain due to fasciitis; Postoperative pain; Radicular and pseudoradicular pain syndromes; Renal colic; Sciatica; Sore throat; Spine pain, acute; Sprain; Stiff neck; Tennis elbow					
Pain due to endoscopic examination					
Wang et al., 1992 (135) (colonoscopy)	100:100	Group comparison	Acupuncture	Standard medication (scopolamine butylbromide, pethidine)	Analgesia was similar in the two groups but there were significantly fewer side-effects in the test group.
Wang et al., 1997 (136) (colonoscopy)	30:29	Randomized controlled trial	Electric acupuncture at zúsānlǐ (ST36) and shàngjùxū (ST37)	Pethidine analgesia	Analgesia was similar in the two groups, but there were fewer side-effects in the test group.
Pain in thromboangiitis obliterans					
Qiu, 1997 (16)	60:30	Group comparison	Body acupuncture (manual)	Medication (intramuscular bucinnazine; also known as bucinperazine)	Effective rates were: • 93.4% in the test group; pain relief started 2–10 min after needling and lasted for 5.6 h • 56.7% in the control group; pain relief started 15–25 min after injection and lasted for 3.1 h.
Periarthritis of shoulder					
Kinoshita, 1973 (38)	15:15	Randomized controlled trial	Acupuncture at specific & basic points	Acupuncture at basic points alone	The therapeutic effect was superior in the test group; the difference was significant.
Shao, 1994 (39)	62:62	Randomized controlled trial	Acupuncture at èrjiān (LI2)	Acupuncture at traditional points	Cure rates were: • 66.1% in the test group after 2.2 treatments • 31.7% in control groups after 8.2 treatments.

Condition/Study	No.	Design	Test group	Control Group	Results
Pertussis, see Whooping cough (pertussis)					
Plantar pain due to fasciitis					
Karen et al., 1991 (*41*)	15 per group	Randomized controlled trial	Acupuncture	Sham acupuncture or conventional sports therapy	True acupuncture produced greater improvement in pain records than conventional sports therapy at the end of the treatment period (4 weeks) and at the end of the follow-up period (3 weeks). There was also a statistically significant difference between true and sham acupuncture.
Polycystic ovary syndrome (Stein–Leventhal syndrome)					
Ma et al., 1996 (*245*)	50:48	Randomized controlled trial	Manual acupuncture plus electric acupuncture plus moxibustion	Conventional Western medication (clomifene)	Clinical cure (assessment of clinical symptoms, ultrasonic examination and radioimmunoassay of sex hormones) was observed in: • 94% of the test group • 62.5% of the control group.
Postextubation in children					
Lee et al., 1998 (*15*)	38:38	Randomized controlled trial	Acupuncture (blood-letting at *shàoshāng* (LU11) at the end of operation)	No acupuncture	If laryngospasm developed, patients were immediately given acupuncture at *shàoshāng* (LU11) or *zhōngfū* (LU1). The laryngospasm was relieved within 1 min in all patients. The incidence of laryngospasm occurring after tracheal extubation in children was: • 5.3% in the test group • 23.7% in the control group.
Postoperative symptoms, closed craniocerebral injury					
Ding et al., 1997 (*252*)	50:50	Randomized controlled trial	Conventional Western medication plus acupuncture	Conventional Western medication (no further details available)	Clinical cure in was observed in: • 13 in the test group; marked improvement in 30; cure and improvement rate, 86% • 7 in the control group; marked improvement in 21; cure and improvement rate, 56%.
Postoperative convalescence					
Xu, 1998 (*101*) (hemiplegia after meningioma removal)	15:15	Group comparison	Body acupuncture	Routine medical treatment (intravenous piracetam)	Improvement of muscular strength and activities after 10 days of treatment was observed in: • 14 in the test group • 8 in the control group.
Postoperative pain					
Christensen et al., 1989 (*72*) (after lower abdominal surgery)	10:10	Randomized controlled trial	Electric acupuncture	No treatment	The pethidine requirements of each patient were recorded. The quantity of pethidine consumed by the test group was half that consumed by the control group.

Acupuncture: review and analysis of controlled clinical trials

Condition/Study	No.	Design	Test group	Control Group	Results
Wang et al., 1990 (76) (after tonsillectomy)	33:33	Group comparison	Acupuncture	Medication (penicillin plus Dobell gargle)	Alleviation of pain, reduction in salivation and speed of wound healing were superior in the test group.
Lü et al., 1993 (74) (after anal surgery)	62:30	Randomized controlled trial	Acupuncture	Bucinnazine	A marked analgesic effect was obtained in: • 77% of the test group • 27% of the control group.
Tsibuliak et al., 1995 (75) (various)	229:91: 229	Group comparison	Acupuncture	Electric stimulation or narcotic analgesics (omnopon (a Chinese opium alkaloid), trimeperidine)	Although less effective than narcotic analgesics, acupuncture provided adequate analgesia in 50% of patients, & noticeably alleviated severity of postoperative complications (nausea, vomiting, retention of urine, intestinal paresis, impaired drainage function of bronchi).
Felhendler et al., 1996 (278) (after knee arthroscopy)	40	Randomized controlled trial	Acupressure (firm pressure across classical acupoints)	Placebo (light pressure in the same area)	60 min and 24 h after treatment, pain scores on a visual analogue scale were lower in the test group.
Chen et al., 1998 (71) (after abdominal hysterectomy or myomectomy)	25 per group	Randomized controlled trial	TENS at zúsānlǐ (ST36) or dermatomal TENS at the level of the surgical incision	Nonacupoint TENS or sham TENS (no electric current)	Peri-incisional dermatomal TENS and TENS at zusanli were equally effective in decreasing postoperative opioid analgesic requirement and in reducing opioid-related side effects. Both of these treatments were more effective than the nonacupoint or sham TENS.
Premenstrual syndrome					
Li et al., 1992 (155)	108:108	Randomized group comparison	Acupuncture	Herbal medication	Total relief of symptoms with no recurrence in 6 months of follow-up was observed in: • 91.7% of the test group • 63% of the control group.
Prostatitis, chronic					
Luo et al., 1994 (149)	100:81	Randomized controlled trial	Acupuncture at zhìbiān (BL54) and sānyīnjiāo (SP6)	Medication (oral sulfamethoxazole)	Relief of symptoms and improvement in sexual function were superior in the test group.
Pruritus, experimentally induced					
Lunderberg et al., 1987 (226)	10	Randomized crossover trial	Manual or electric acupuncture	Placebo acupuncture (superficial insertion of needle with no specific sensation)	Acupuncture and electric acupuncture reduced subjective itch intensity more effectively than placebo acupuncture. The difference was significant. The results suggest that the two test procedures could be tried in clinical conditions associated with pruritus.

Condition/Study	No.	Design	Test group	Control Group	Results
Pulmonary heart disease, chronic					
Zou et al., 1998 (279)	30:29	Randomized controlled trial	Ginger moxibustion plus acupoint injection	Routine Western treatment (oxygen inhalation, antibiotics and bronchodilators)	After 1.5–2 months of treatment, improvement was observed in: • 27/30 (90%) of the test group; in 1-year follow-up, acute respiratory infection occurred in 7 • 12/29 (41.4%) of the control group; in 1-year follow-up, acute respiratory infection occurred in 26.
Radicular and pseudoradicular pain syndromes					
Krecczi et al., 1986 (57)	21	Randomized single-blind crossover trial	Laser acupuncture	Mock laser acupuncture	Laser acupuncture was more effective than placebo in 20 out of 21 patients.
Raynaud syndrome, primary					
Appiah et al., 1997 (244)	17:16	Randomized controlled trial	Acupuncture	No treatment	Mean duration of the capillary flowstop reaction induced by local cooling test decreased from 71 s to 24 s (week 1 compared to week 12, $P = 0.001$) in test group. Changes in control group weren't significant. Authors concluded that Chinese acupuncture is a reasonable alternative in treating patients with primary Raynaud syndrome. There was a significant decrease in the frequency of attacks by: 63% in the test group and 27% in the control group.
Recurrent lower urinary-tract infection					
Aune et al., 1998 (152)	67	Randomized controlled trial	Acupuncture	Sham acupuncture or no treatment	Proportions remaining free of lower urinary-tract infection during 6-month observation period were: • 85% in the acupuncture group • 58% in the sham acupuncture group • 36% in the untreated group.
Reflex sympathetic dystrophy					
Kho, 1995 (280)	28	Double-blind placebo-controlled trial	Acupuncture	Sham acupuncture	Acupuncture was beneficial.
Renal colic					
Lee et al., 1992 (65)	22:16	Randomized controlled trial	Acupuncture	Medication (injection of a metamizole–camylofin combination)	Both groups experienced a significant decrease in pain levels, with the acupuncture group improving slightly more. Side-effects occurred in: • 0/22 in the test group • 7/16 in the control group.

Acupuncture: review and analysis of controlled clinical trials

Condition/Study	No.	Design	Test group	Control Group	Results
Zhang et al., 1992 (7)	126:118	Group comparison	Acupuncture	Medication (injection of atropine plus pethidine)	An analgesic effect was observed in: • 99.2% of the test group • 71.2% of the control group.
Li et al., 1993 (66)	25:27	Randomized controlled trial	Acupuncture	Medication (injection of atropine plus promethazine and bucinnazine)	Relief of pain was observed in: • all patients in the test group in 25 min on average • 90% of the patients in the control group in 50 min.
Retention of urine, traumatic					
Pan et al., 1996 (146)	76:32	Randomized controlled trial	Acupuncture	Medication (intramuscular neostigmine bromide)	The therapeutic effect of acupuncture was markedly superior to that of neostigmine injection.
Retinopathy, central serous					
Yu et al., 1997 (281)	83:135	Group comparison	Acupuncture (manual)	Medication (rutoside, vitamin C, troxerutin)	Cure rates were: • 46/86 (49.5%) eyes in test group; average duration of treatment required, 50.6 days • 52/146 (35.6%) eyes in control group; average duration of treatment required, 63.6 days.
Rheumatoid arthritis					
Man et al., 1974 (4)	10:10	Group comparison	Electric acupuncture	Sham acupuncture	Pain relief was observed in: • 90% of the treatment group • 10% of the control group.
Ruchkin et al., 1987 (5)	10:6	Double-blind controlled trial	Auricular electric-acupuncture	Sham electric acupuncture (no electrical stimulation)	Subjective improvement was observed in: • all patients in the test group • 1 patient in the control group.
Sun et al., 1992 (6)	378:56	Group comparison	Warming acupuncture	Acupuncture	Marked improvement was observed in: • 65.5% of the test group • 26.8% of the control group.
Schizophrenia					
Jia et al., 1986 (195)	24:13	Controlled trial	Laser acupuncture	Medication (chlorpromazine)	After 6 weeks of treatment, marked improvement was observed in: • 78% of the test group • 39% of the control group.
Zhang et al., 1994 (282)	38:31	Randomized controlled trial	Electric acupuncture plus conventional medication (various)	Conventional medication (various)	The therapeutic effect was significantly greater in the test group.

4. Summary table of controlled clinical trials

Condition/Study	No.	Design	Test group	Control Group	Results
Sciatica					
Kinoshita, 1971 (50)	15:15	Randomized controlled trial	Acupuncture with deep insertion of needles (10–30 mm)	Acupuncture with superficial puncture (5 mm)	The therapeutic effect was greater in the test group. The difference was statistically significant.
Kinoshita, 1981 (51)	15:15	Randomized controlled trial	Acupuncture at dàchángshū (BL25) with deep puncture (6 cm)	Acupuncture with superficial puncture (2 cm)	The therapeutic effect on tenderness, Lasegue's sign, and subjective symptoms was greater in the test group. The difference was significant.
Shen, 1987 (53)	50:50	Group comparison	Long-needle acupuncture	Classical acupuncture	Effective rates were: • 96% of the test group • 72% of the control group.
Li, 1991 (52)	100:70	Group comparison	Acupuncture at xiazhibian	Acupuncture at zhibiān (BL54)	Effective rates were: • 98% of test group after 15.8 treatments, on average • 81.4% of the control group after 27.7 treatments.
Sexual dysfunction, see Defective ejaculation; Male sexual dysfunction, non-organic					
Sialorrhoea, antipsychotic-induced					
Xiong et al., 1993 (242)	60:60	Randomized controlled trial	Acupuncture	Anisodamine	After 10 days of treatment, marked reduction in salivation was achieved in: • 96.7% of the test group • 35.9% of the control group.
Simple obesity in children					
Yu et al., 1998 (283)	101:101:50	Randomized controlled trial	Photo-acupuncture or auricular acupressure	No treatment	The effects of photo-acupuncture and auricular acupressure were satisfactory, with better results for the former. After 3 months of acupuncture treatment, the obesity indices decreased significantly and levels of blood lipids, glucose, hydrocortisone and triiodothyronine were all markedly improved.
Sjögren syndrome					
List et al., 1998 (243)	21	Randomized controlled trial	Acupuncture	No treatment	A significant increase in paraffin-stimulated saliva secretion was found in both groups. There were no statistically significant differences in unstimulated salivary secretion between groups. The study showed that acupuncture is of limited value for patients with primary Sjögren syndrome.

Acupuncture: review and analysis of controlled clinical trials

Condition/Study	No.	Design	Test group	Control Group	Results
Small airway obstruction					
Chen et al., 1997 (284)	21:21:21	Randomized controlled trial	Body acupuncture (40 min)	Body acupuncture (20 min and 60 min)	Small airway function in bronchial asthma and chronic bronchitis improved in all three groups. The best result was obtained in the test group.
Smoking, see Dependence, tobacco					
Sore throat (see also Tonsillitis, acute)					
Gunsberger, 1973 (118)	100 per group	Group comparison	Acupuncture at a single point or at 2 points	No treatment (acupuncture refusers) or petroleum jelly placebo	Results in the two treatment groups were significantly better than in the two control groups. At 48 h, 90% of those receiving acupuncture at 2 points were still reporting pain relief compared with only 30% of those receiving no treatment.
Spine pain, acute (see also Low back pain; Sciatica)					
Santiesteban, 1984 (285)	5:5	Randomized controlled trial	Electric acupuncture	Selected physical therapy	The test group showed significant increases in range of motion, straight leg raising, & decreased pain immediately after treatment. Control group showed no improvement.
Sprain					
Jiao, 1991 (68) (limb)	200:100	Randomized controlled trial	Acupuncture	Physiotherapy	Pain was relieved after 1 session of treatment in: • 32% of the test group (in 84% after 9 sessions) • 0% of the control group (in 18% after 9 sessions).
Jin, 1991 (69) (lumbar)	346:50	Group comparison	Hand acupuncture	Medication (analgesic)	Pain was relieved and function restored in: • 1–3 days (average 1.06 days) in test group • 3–10 days (average 4.38 days) in control group.
Zheng, 1997 (70) (lumbar)	100:50	Randomized group comparison	Hand acupuncture	Body acupuncture	Cure (disappearance of symptoms, free movement of the lower back, and no recurrence in 3 years) immediately after 1 session of treatment in: • 82.4% of the test group • 52.9% of the control group.
Stiff neck					
Wu, 1997 (286)	100:32	Group comparison	Acupuncture at *laozhen*	Medication (ibuprofen 0.3 g, 3 times per day)	Cure was observed in: • 80/100 (80%) in the test group after the first session, 10 after the second, and 4 after the third; 6 did not respond in 3 days • 12/32 (38%) in the control group on the first day, 6 on the second, and 2 on the third; 12 did not respond in 3 days.

Condition/Study	No.	Design	Test group	Control Group	Results
Stroke					
Chen et al., 1990 (89) (ischaemic))	20 per group	Randomized controlled trial	Acupuncture	Medication (mannitol, dextrose, citicoline)	A better therapeutic effect (as assessed by EEG-map and somatosensory-evoked potential) was observed in the test group.
Zou et al., 1990 (287) (ischaemic)	32:31	Randomized controlled trial	Acupuncture	Medication (vinpocetine)	A better therapeutic effect was observed in the test group.
Bai et al., 1993 (88) (ischaemic)	40 per group	Randomized controlled trial	Acupuncture	Medication Beniol (a Chinese medicine containing linoleic acid, inositol & other vitamins), troxerutin, nimodipine)	A better neurological outcome was observed in the test group.
Hu et al., 1993 (94) (ischaemic)	30:30	Randomized controlled trial	Physiotherapy plus acupuncture	Physiotherapy	A better neurological outcome was observed for physiotherapy plus acupuncture than for physiotherapy alone.
Jin et al., 1993 (99) (hemiplegia after stroke)	108:100	Randomized group comparison	Temporal acupuncture	Traditional body acupuncture	Significantly better results were obtained in the test group.
Liang, 1993 (100) (sequelae of stroke)	50:50	Randomized controlled trial	Temporal acupuncture	Traditional body acupuncture	Significantly better results were obtained in the test group.
Johansson et al., 1993 (95) (sequelae of stroke)	38:40	Randomized controlled trial	Acupuncture plus physiotherapy and occupational therapy	Physiotherapy and occupational therapy	A more rapid and more complete recovery was observed in the test group.
Zhang et al.,1994 (102) (stroke with aphasia)	22:22	Randomized controlled trial	Scalp electric acupuncture	No treatment	A more rapid and more complete recovery observed in the test group.
Liao, 1997 (91) (hemiplegia after stroke)	108:107	Group comparison	Acupuncture at shŏusānlĭ (LI10) and fútù (ST32)	Routine medication plus hyperbaric oxygenation	Marked improvement after 20 days of treatment was observed in: • 66.7% of the test group • 29.0% of the control group.

Acupuncture: review and analysis of controlled clinical trials

Condition/Study	No.	Design	Test group	Control Group	Results
Jiang et al., 1997 (90) (spontaneous limb pain after stroke)	30:30	Randomized controlled trial	Electric acupuncture	Conventional Western medication (carbamazepine)	After 30 days of treatment, the two groups showed similar amelioration of pain. Effective rates were: • 90% in the test group • 86.7% in the control group.
Liu et al., 1997 (92) (myodynamia after stroke)	78:56:30	Group comparison	Scalp or body acupuncture	Medication	Functional recovery was observed in: • 75.6% of the scalp acupuncture group; total effective rate 98.7% • 51.8% of the body acupuncture group; total effective rate 92.8% • 16.7% control group; total effective rate 80%.
Kjendahl et al., 1997 (97) (subacute stroke)	21:20	Randomized controlled trial	Rehabilitation programme plus acupuncture	Rehabilitation programme	The test group improved significantly more than the control group during the treatment period of 6 weeks, and even more during the following year, according to motor-assessment scale, ADL, Nottingham health profile and social situation.
Gosman-Hedstrom et al., 1998 (96) (acute stroke)	104	Randomized controlled trial	Conventional rehabilitation plus deep acupuncture	Conventional rehabilitation plus superficial acupuncture or conventional rehabilitation alone	There were no differences between the groups in respect of changes in the neurological score and the Barthel and Sunnaas activities of daily living index scores after 3 and 12 months.
Si et al., 1998 (93) (acute ischaemic stroke)	42	Randomized controlled trial	Electric acupuncture plus medication	Medication	Clinical functional recovery was significantly better in the test group.
Wong et al., 1999 (98) (hemiplegia after stroke)	59:59	Randomized controlled trial	Electric acupuncture plus rehabilitation	Rehabilitation	Patients in the test group had a shorter hospital stay for rehabilitation and better neurological and functional outcomes than those in the control group, with a significant difference in scores for self-care and locomotion.
Temporomandibular joint dysfunction (see also Facial pain, including craniomandibular disorders)					
Raustia et al., 1986 (288)	25:25	Randomized controlled trial	Acupuncture	Standard stomatognathic treatment	Both treatments resulted in a significant reduction in symptoms and signs. Acupuncture seems to be useful as a complementary treatment, especially in cases with evidence of physiological or neuromuscular disturbances.

4. Summary table of controlled clinical trials

Condition/Study	No.	Design	Test group	Control Group	Results
Tennis elbow Brattberg, 1983 (42)	34:26	Group comparison	Acupuncture	Steroid injection	Improvement was observed at follow-up in: • 61.8% of the test group • 30.8% of the control group.
Haker et al., 1990 (43)	44:38	Randomized group comparison	Classical acupuncture	Superficial acupuncture	Short-term improvement was significantly greater in the test group.
Molsberger et al., 1994 (44)	24:24	Placebo-controlled, single-blind trial with independent evaluation	Acupuncture	Placebo (acupuncture, avoiding penetration of the skin)	Pain relief of at least 50% after 1 treatment was reported by: • 19 of the test group; average duration of analgesia after 1 treatment, 20.2 h • 6 of the control group; average duration of analgesia after 1 treatment, 1.4 h.
Tietze syndrome Yang, 1997 (246)	108:64	Group comparison	Acupuncture (manual) plus cupping	Routine medication (oral indometacin and local injection of prednisolone or procaine) plus physiotherapy	After 3 weeks of treatment, cure was observed in: • 70/108 (64.8%) in the test group • 24/64 (37.5%) in the control group.
Tinnitus Jin et al., 1998 (220) (subjective)	35:35	Randomized controlled trial	Body acupuncture	Routine medication, including anisodamine	After 6 weeks of treatment cure was observed in: • 8 (22.9%) in the test group; 10 (28.6%) markedly improved • 2 (5.7%) in the control group; 6 (17.1%) markedly improved.
Vilholm et al., 1998 (221) (severe)	54	Randomized controlled crossover trial	Body acupuncture	Placebo	There was no statistically significant difference between the two groups.
Tonsillitis, acute Chen, 1987 (117)	220:50	Group comparison	Acupuncture	Antibiotics (penicillin, etc.)	Earlier relief of fever and sore throat was observed in the test group.
Tourette syndrome Tian et al., 1996 (217)	68:17	Randomized controlled trial	Body acupuncture plus auricular acupressure	Conventional Western medication (haloperidol)	Cure was observed in: • 30.9% of the test group; effective rate at 6-month follow-up, 46/57 (89.7%) • 11.8% of the control group; effective rate at 6-month follow-up, 5/13 (69.7%) in the control group.

Acupuncture: review and analysis of controlled clinical trials

Condition/Study	No.	Design	Test group	Control Group	Results
Jin, 1998 (216)	30:30	Randomized controlled trial	Body acupuncture plus auricular acupressure	Conventional Western medication (haloperidol)	After 1 month of treatment, clinical cure with no recurrence at 6-month follow-up in: • 30.0% of test group; overall effective rate 93.4% • 6.7% of control group; overall effective rate 76.7%.
Ulcerative colitis, chronic					
Wu et al., 1995 (134)	24:11	Group comparison	Moxibustion with herbal partition	Sulfasalazine	After 3 months of treatment, clinical cure was observed in: • 13/24 (54%) in test group; improvement in 10 • 3/11 (27%) in the control group; improvement in 4. The difference was significant.
Ma et al., 1997 (289)	60:30	Randomized controlled trial	Body acupuncture plus moxibustion.	Sulfasalazine plus metronidazole	After 30 days of treatment, cure (assessed both clinically and endoscopically) was observed in: • 76.7% of the test group • 56.7% of the control group.
Urinary tract problems, see Female urethral syndrome; Neuropathic bladder in spinal cord injury; Recurrent lower urinary tract infection; Renal colic; Urolithiasis					
Urolithiasis					
Zhang et al., 1992 (7)	126:118	Group comparison	Acupuncture	Fluid infusion plus herbal medication)	Cure (elimination of symptoms and signs and no residual stones revealed by X-ray or ultrasound examination) was observed in: • 90.48% of the test group • 33.05% of the control group.
Vascular dementia					
Lai, 1997 (290)	30:30	Randomized controlled trial	Manual plus electric acupuncture	Aniracetam	Improvement after 6 weeks of treatment was observed in: • 26 (86.7%) of the test group • 19 (63.3%) of the control group.
Liu et al., 1998 (291)	60:60: 30:30	Randomized controlled trial	(1) Scalp electric acupuncture	(2) Nimodipine, (3) Electric acupuncture plus medication (nimodipine), or (4) No treatment	Assessment by various neuropsychological scales showed that effects of test & control procedures were comparable. After 8 weeks of treatment, assessment (of memory, intelligence and ability to take care of oneself) showed improvement in: • 68.3% of group (1) • 71.6% of group (2) • 73.3% of group (3) • 23.3% of group (4).

Condition/Study	No.	Design	Test group	Control Group	Results
Jiang et al., 1998 (292)	33:33	Randomized controlled trial	Electric acupuncture	Dihydroergotoxine	Results were superior in the test group, as assessed by the Hasegawa dementia scale and functional activities questionnaire, increase in superoxide dismutase and decreases in lipid peroxide and nitric oxide.
Viral encephalitis in children, late stage					
Wang, 1998 (293)	72:42	Group comparison	Scalp electric and manual acupuncture plus routine medication as for control group	Routine medication (including antiviral and anti-inflammatory agents, and nutrients for brain tissue)	Effective rates were: • 59/72 (81.9%) in the test group • 19/42 (45.2%) in the control group.
Whooping cough (pertussis)					
Yao et al., 1996 (87)	145:50	Randomized controlled trial	Acupuncture at *bāxié* (EX-UE9)	Chloramphenicol intravenous drip	After 7 days of treatment, cure was observed in: • 98.6% of the test group • 10% of the control group.

References

1.   Lewith GT et al. On the evaluation of the clinical effect of acupuncture. *Pain*, 1983, **16**:111 – 127.

2.   Pomeranz B. Acupuncture analgesia for chronic pain: brief survey of clinical trials. In: Pomeranz B, Stux G, eds. *Scientific bases of acupuncture*. Berlin/Heidelberg, Springer-Verlag, 1989: 197 – 199.

3.   Richardson PH et al. Acupuncture for the treatment of pain—a review of evaluation research. *Pain*, 1986, **24**:15 – 40.

4.   Man SC et al. Preliminary clinical study of acupuncture in rheumatoid arthritis. *Journal of Rheumatology*, 1974, **1**:126 – 129.

5.   Ruchkin IN et al. [Auriculo-electropuncture in rheumatoid arthritis (a double-blind study).] *Terapevticheskii Arkhiv*, 1987, **59**(12):26 – 30 [in Russian].

6.   Sun LQ et al. [Observation of the effect of acupuncture and moxibustion on rheumatoid arthritis in 434 cases.] *Chinese Acupuncture and Moxibustion*, 1992, **12**(1):9 – 11 [in Chinese].

7.   Zhang WR et al. [Clinical observation of acupuncture in treating kidney and ureter stones.] *Chinese Acupuncture and Moxibustion*, 1992, **12**(3):5 – 6 [in Chinese].

8.   Li KR. [Analysis on the effect of acupuncture treatment in 1383 adults with bacillary dysentery.] *Chinese Acupuncture and Moxibustion*, 1990, **10**(4):113 – 114 [in Chinese].

9.   Qiu ML et al. [A clinical study on acupuncture treatment of acute bacillary dysentery.] In: Zhang XT, ed. [*Researches on acupuncture-moxibustion and acupuncture-anaesthesia.*] Beijing, Science Press, 1986: 567 – 572 [in Chinese].

10. Yu SZ et al. Clinical observation of 162 cases of acute bacillary dysentery treated by acupuncture. *World Journal of Acupuncture-Moxibustion*, 1992, **2**(3):13 – 14.

11. Zhang XP. [Researches on the mechanism of acupuncture and moxibustion.] Anhui, Anhui Science and Technology Press, 1983 [in Chinese.]

12. Stux G, Pomeranz B. *Acupuncture —textbook and atlas*. Berlin: Springer-Verlag, 1987: 18 – 19.

13. Lewith GT et al. On the evaluation of the clinical effects of acupuncture: a problem reassessed and a framework for future research. *Journal of Alternative and Complementary Medicine*, 1996, **2**(1):79 – 90.

14. Shen SJ. [Immediate analgesic effect of acupuncture at binao (LI 14) for pain due to subconjunctival injection.] *Chinese Acupuncture and Moxibustion*, 1996, **16**(2):71 – 72 [in Chinese].

15. Lee CK et al. The effect of acupuncture on the incidence of postextubation laryngospasm in children. *Anaesthesia*, 1998, **53**(9):917–920.

16. Qiu L. [Acupuncture treatment of severe leg pain in 60 cases of thromboangitis obliterans.] *Chinese Acupuncture and Moxibustion*, 1997, **17**(11):677 – 678 [in Chinese].

17. Ahonen E et al. Acupuncture and physiotherapy in the treatment of myogenic headache patients: pain relief and EMG activity. *Advances in Pain Research and Therapy*, 1983, **5**:571 – 576.

18. Chen XS et al. [Observation of penetrating acupuncture treatment of migraine in 45 cases.] *Shanxi Journal of Traditional Chinese Medicine*, 1997, **13**(6):32 – 33 [in Chinese].

19. **Doerr-Proske H et al.** [A muscle and vascular oriented relaxation program for the treatment of chronic migraine patients. A randomized clinical control groups study on the effectiveness of a biobehavioural treatment program]. *Zeitschrift für Psychosomatische Medizin und Psychoanalyse*, 1985, 31(3):247 – 266 [in German].

20. **Dowson DI et al.** The effects of acupuncture versus placebo in the treatment of headache. *Pain*, 1985, **21**:35 – 42.

21. **Kubiena G et al.** Akupunktur bei Migräne. [Acupuncture treatment of migraine.] *Deutsche Zeitschrift für Akunpunktur*, 1992, **35**(6):140 – 148 [in German].

22. **Liu AS et al.** ["Three Scalp Needles" in the treatment of migraine.] *New Tradiitional Chinese Medicine*, 1997, **29**(4) 25 – 26 [in Chinese].

23. **Loh L et al.** Acupuncture versus medical treatment for migraine and muscle tension headaches. *Journal of Neurology, Neurosurgery and Psychiatry*, 1984, **47**:333 – 337.

24. **Tavola T et al.** Traditional Chinese acupuncture in the treatment of tension-type headache: a controlled study. *Pain*, 1992, **48**:325 – 329.

25. **Vincent CA.** A controlled trial of the treatment of migraine by acupuncture. *Clinical Journal of Pain*, 1989, **5**:305 – 312.

26. **Weinschütz T et al.** Zur neuroregulativen Wirkung der Akupunktur bei Kopfschmerzpatienten. [Neuroregulatory action of acupuncture in headache patients.] *Deutsche Zeitschrift für Akupunktur*, 1994, **37**(5):106 – 117 [in German].

27. **Xu Z et al.** [Treatment of migraine by qi-manipulating acupuncture.] *Shanghai Journal of Acupuncture and Moxibustion*, 1993, **12**(3):97 – 100 [in Chinese].

28. **Cai L.** [Observation of therapeutic effects of intractable prosopodynia treated by retaining the filiform needle for long time.] *Chinese Acupuncture and Moxibustion*, 1996, **16**(4):190 – 191 [in Chinese].

29. **Hansen PE et al.** Acupuncture treatment of chronic facial pain: a controlled crossover trial. *Headache*, 1983, **23**:66 – 69.

30. **Johansson A et al.** Acupuncture for the treatment of facial muscular pain. *Acta Odontologica Scandinavica*, 1991, **49**:153 – 158.

31. **List T.** Acupuncture in the treatment of patients with craniomandibular disorders: comparative, longitudinal and methodological studies. *Swedish Dental Journal*, 1992, 87(Suppl. 1):1–159.

32. **Pohjola RT et al.** Rationale behind acupuncture treatment of temporomandibular joint dysfunction. *Akupunktur Theorie und Praxis*, 1986, **14**(4):263.

33. **Birch S et al.** Controlled trial of Japanese acupuncture for chronic myofascial neck pain: assessment of specific and nonspecific effects of treatment. *Clinical Journal of Pain*, 1998, **14**(3):248–255.

34. **David J et al.** Chronic neck pain: a comparison of acupuncture treatment and physiotherapy. *British Journal of Rheumatology*, 1998, **37**(10):1118–1132.

35. **Coan R et al.** The acupuncture treatment of neck pain: a randomized controlled study. *American Journal of Chinese Medicine*, 1982, **9**:326 – 332.

36. **Loy TT.** Treatment of cervical spondylosis: electro-acupuncture versus physiotherapy. *Medical Journal of Australia*, 1983, **2**:32 – 34.

37. **Petrie JP et al.** A controlled study of acupuncture in neck pain. *British Journal of Rheumatology*, 1986, **25**:271 – 275.

38. **Kinoshita H.** [Effect of specific treatment for periarthritis of shoulder.] *Journal of the Japanese Acupuncture and Moxibustion Society*, 1973, **22**(1):23 – 28. [in Japanese].

39. **Shao CJ.** [Treatment of 62 cases of periarthritis of shoulder by needling at LI 2.] *Chinese Acupuncture and Moxibustion*, 1994, **14**(5):247 – 248 [in Chinese].

40. **Deluze C et al.** Electroacupuncture in fibromyalgia: result of a controlled trial. *British Medical Journal*, 1992, **305**:1249 – 1252.

41. **Karen D et al.** True acupuncture vs. sham acupuncture and conventional sports medicine therapy for plantar fasciitis pain: a controlled, double blind study. *International Journal of Clinical Acupuncture*, 1991, 2(3):247 – 253.

42. **Brattberg G.** Acupuncture therapy for tennis elbow. *Pain*, 1983, **16**:285 – 288.

43. **Haker E et al.** Acupuncture treatment in epicondylalgia: a comparison study of two acupuncture techniques. *Clinical Journal of Pain*, 1990, **6**:221 – 226.

44. **Molsberger A et al.** The analgesic effect of acupuncture in chronic tennis elbow pain. *British Journal of Rheumatology*, 1994, **33**(12):1162 – 1165.

45. **Coan R et al.** The acupuncture treatment of low back pain: a randomized controlled treatment. *American Journal of Chinese Medicine*, 1980, **8**:181 – 189.

46. **Gunn CC et al.** Dry needling of muscle motor points for chronic low-back pain. *Spine*, 1980, **5**(3):279 – 291.

47. **Lehmann TR et al.** Efficacy of electroacupuncture and TENS in the rehabilitation of chronic low back pain patients. *Pain*, 1986, **26**:277 – 290.

48. **MacDonald AJR et al.** Superficial acupuncture in the relief of chronic low back pain. *Annals of the Royal College of Surgeons of England*, 1983, **65**:44 – 46.

49. **Mendelson G et al.** Acupuncture treatment of low back pain: a double-blind placebo-controlled trial. *American Journal of Medicine*, 1983, **74**:49 – 55.

50. **Kinoshita H.** [Clinical trials on reinforcing and reducing manipulations.] *Journal of the Japanese Acupuncture and Moxibustion Society*, 1971, **20**(3):6 – 13 [in Japanese].

51. **Kinoshita H.** [Clinical research in the use of paraneural acupuncture for sciatica.] *Journal of the Japanese Acupuncture and Moxibustion Society*, 1981, **30**(1):4 – 13 [in Japanese].

52. **Li HY.** [Controlled study of 170 cases of sciatica treated with acupuncture at the lower zhibian point.] *Chinese Acupuncture and Moxibustion*, 1991, **11**(5):17 – 18 [in Chinese].

53. **Shen GZ.** [Treatment of 100 cases of sciatica by applying the long needle.] *Chinese Acupuncture and Moxibustion*, 1987, **7**(2):77 [in Chinese].

54. **Christensen BV et al.** Acupuncture treatment of severe knee osteoarthrosis: a long-term study. *Acta Anaesthesiologica Scandinavica*, 1992, **36**:519 – 25 (also i*Ugeskrift for Laeger*, 1993, **155**(49):4007 – 4011 [in Danish]).

55. **Junnila SYT.** Acupuncture superior to piroxicam in the treatment of osteoarthritis. *American Journal of Acupuncture*, 1982, **10**:341 – 345.

56. **Maruno A.** [Comparative analysis of electrical acupuncture therapy for arthrosis of the knee.] *Journal of the Japanese Acupuncture and Moxibustion Society*, 1976, **25**(3):52 – 54 [in Japanese].

57. **Kreczi T et al.** A comparison of laser acupuncture versus placebo in radicular and pseudoradicular pain syndromes as recorded by subjective responses of patients. *Acupunture and Electrotherapy Research*, 1986, **11**:207 – 216.

58. **Berman BM et al.** A randomized trial of acupuncture as an adjunctive therapy in osteoarthritis of the knee. *Rheumatology*, 1999, **38**(4):346–354.

59. **Xiao J et al.** [Analysis of the therapeutic effect on 41 cases of rheumatoid arthritis treated by acupuncture and the influence on interleukin-2.] *Chinese Acupuncture and Moxibustion*, 1992, **12**(6):306 – 308 [in Chinese].

60. **Li ZW et al.** [Controlled study of gouty arthritis treated with blood-pricking acupuncture.] *Chinese Acupuncture and Moxibustion*, 1993, **13**(4):179 – 182 [in Chinese].

61. **Pan HL.** [Observation of 39 cases of gout treated with plum-blossom needling plus cupping.] *Zhenjiu Linchuang Zazhi*, 1997, **13**(3):29 [in Chinese].

62. **Mo TW.** [Observation of 70 cases of biliary ascariasis treated by acupuncture.] *Chinese Acupuncture and Moxibustion*, 1987, **7**(5):237 – 238 [in Chinese].

63. **Wu XL et al.** Observation of acupuncture treatment of biliary colic in 142 cases. *Journal of Acupuncture-Moxibustion*, 1992, **8**(6):8.

64. **Yang TG et al.** [Clinical report of electro-acupuncture analgesia in the treatment of abdominal colics.] *Jiangsu Journal of Traditional Chinese Medicine*, 1990, **11**(12):31 [in Chinese].

65. **Lee YH et al.** Acupuncture in the treatment of renal colic. *Journal of Urology*, 1992, **147**:16 – 18.

66. **Li JX et al.** [Observation of the therapeutic effect of acupuncture treatment of renal colic.] *Chinese Acupuncture and Moxibustion*, 1993, **13**(2):65 – 66 [in Chinese].

67. **Shu X, et al.** [Observation of acupuncture treatment of abdominal pain in acute gastroenteritis.] *Chinese Acupuncture and Moxibustion*, 1997, **17**(11):653 – 654 [in Chinese].

68. **Jiao Y.** Acupuncture analgesia in treating sprain of limbs. *Acupuncture Research*, 1991, **11**(3 – 4):253 – 254.

69. **Jin CL.** [Clinical observation of 346 cases of acute lumbar sprain treated with hand-acupuncture.] *Chinese Acupuncture and Moxibustion*, 1991, **11**(3):30 [in Chinese].

70. **Zheng LM.** [Hand acupuncture treatment of 100 cases of acute lumbar sprain.] *Chinese Acupuncture and Moxibustion*, 1997, **17**(4):201 – 202 [in Chinese].

71. **Chen L et al.** The effect of location of transcutaneous electrical nerve stimulation of postoperative opioid analgesic requirement: acupoint versus nonacupoint stimulation. *Anesthesia and Analgesia*, 1998, **87**(5):1129–1134.

72. **Christensen PA et al.** Electroacupuncture and postoperative pain. *British Journal of Anaesthesia*, 1989, **62**:258 – 262.

73. **Lao L et al.** Evaluation of acupuncture for pain control after oral surgery: a placebo-controlled trial. *Archives of Otolaryngology, Head and Neck Surgery*, 1999, **125**(5):567–572.

74. **Lü D et al.** [Observation of the analgesic effect of acupuncture for pain after anal surgery.] *Shanghai Journal of Acupuncture-Moxibustion*, 1993, **12**(2):72 [in Chinese].

75. **Tsibuliak VN et al.** [Acupuncture analgesia and analgesic transcutaneous electroneurostimulation in the early postoperative period.] *Anesteziologiia i Reanimatologiia*, 1995, (2):93 – 97 [in Russian].

76. **Wang Q et al.** [Acupuncture treatment of post-tonsillectomy pain in 33 cases.] *Chinese Journal of Integrated Traditional and Western Medicine*, 1990, **10**(4):244 – 245 [in Chinese].

77. **Lao LX et al.** Efficacy of Chinese acupuncture on postoperative oral surgery pain. *Oral Surgery, Oral Medicine, Oral Pathology, Oral Radiology and Endodontics*, 1995, **79**(4):423 – 428.

78. **Sung YF et al.** Comparison of the effects of acupuncture and codeine on postoperative dental pain. *Anesthesia and Analgesia*, 1977, **56**:473 – 478.

79. **Zheng J et al.** [Prevention and treatment of pain caused by pulp devitalisation with arsenical.] *Journal of the Zhejiang College of Traditional Chinese Medicine*, 1990, **14**(6):6 [in Chinese].

80. **Sukandar SD et al.** [Analgesic effect of acupuncture in acute periodontitis apicalis.] *Cermin Dunia Kedokteran*, 1995, (105):5 – 10 [in Indonesian]

81. **Rosted P.** The use of acupuncture in dentistry: a systematic review. *Acupuncture-Medicine*, 1998, **16**(1):43–48.

82. **Zhang YF et al.** [Clinical observation of acupuncture painless labour in 150 cases.] *Chinese Acupuncture and Moxibustion*, 1995, **15**(4):182 – 183 [in Chinese].

83. **Qian XZ.** [Achievements in scientific studies on acupuncture-moxibustion and acupuncture-anaesthesia in China.] In: Zhang XT, ed. [*Researches on acupuncture-moxibustion and acupuncture-anaesthesia.*] Beijing, Science Press, 1986: 1 – 13 [in Chinese].

84. **Xu BQ et al.** [Experimental studies on acupuncture treatment of acute bacillary dysentery—the role of humoral immune mechanism.] In: Zhang XT, ed. [*Researches on acupuncture-moxibustion and acupuncture-anaesthesia.*]Beijing, Science Press, 1986: 573 – 578 [in Chinese].

85. **Wang XY et al.** Acupuncture and moxibustion in the treatment of asymptomatic hepatitis B virus carriers by strengthening the body resistance to eliminate pathogenic factors: a clinical experimental study. *International Journal of Clinical Acupuncture*, 1991, **2**(2):117 – 125.

86. **Song XG et al.** The effect of moxibustion on the kidney function of the patients with epidemic haemorrhagic fever. *World Journal of Acupuncture-Moxibustion*, 1992, **2**(1):17 – 19.

87. **Yao HH et al.** [Clinical study on treatment of pertussis with acupuncture at baxie (EX:E9).] *Chinese Acupuncture and Moxibustion*, 1996, **16**(11):604 [in Chinese].

88. **Bai XY et al.** [A comparative study of acupuncture and Western medicine in the treatment of stroke]. *Chinese Acupuncture and Moxibustion*, 1993, **13**(1):1 – 4 [in Chinese].

89. **Chen DZ et al.** [Evaluation of therapeutic effects of acupuncture in treating ischaemic cerebrovascular disease.] *Chinese Journal of Integrated Traditional and Western Medicine*, 1990, **10**(9):526 – 528 [in Chinese].

90. **Jiang ZY et al.** [Clinical study on needling jiaji (EX – B2) in the treatment of thalamic spontaneous pain induced by stroke.] *Journal of Traditional Chinese Medicine*, 1997, **38**(10):599 – 601 [in Chinese].

91. **Liao SH.** [Treatment of stroke with talon needling at LI10 and ST32.] *Chinese Acupuncture and Moxibustion*, 1997, **17**(8):479 – 480 [in Chinese].

92. **Liu YJ et al.** Needling scalp points in treating cerebrovascular diseases: a report of 78 cases. *International Journal of Clinical Acupuncture*, 1997, **8**(3):231–234.

93. **Si QM et al.** Effects of electroacupuncture on acute cerebral infarction. *Acupuncture and Electro-Therapeutics Research*, 1998, **23**(2):117–124.

94. **Hu HH et al.** A randomized controlled trial on the treatment for acute partial ischemic stroke with acupuncture. *Neuroepidemiology*, 1993, **12**:106 – 113.

95. **Johansson K et al.** Can sensory stimulation improve the functional outcome in stroke patients? *Neurology*, 1993, **43**:2189 – 2192.

96. **Gosman-Hedstrom G et al.** Effects of acupuncture treatment on daily life activities and quality of life: a controlled, prospective, and randomized study of acute stroke patients. *Stroke*, 1998, **29**(10):2100–2108.

97. **Kjendahl A et al.** A one year follow-up study on the effects of acupuncture in the treatment of stroke patients in the subacute stage: a randomized, controlled study. *Clinical Rehabilitation*, 1997, **11**(3):192–200.

98. **Wong AM et al.** Clinical trial of electrical acupuncture on hemiplegic stroke patients. *American Journal of Physical Medicine and Rehabilitation*, 1999, **78**(2):117–122.

99. **Jin R et al.** [Clinical observation of temporal needling in the treatment of postapoplectic sequelae.] *Chinese Acupuncture and Moxibustion*, 1993, **13**(1):11 – 12. [in Chinese].

100. **Liang RA.** Clinical observation and experimental studies on the treatment of sequelae of stroke by needling temporal points. *International Journal of Clinical Acupuncture*, 1993, **4**(1):19 – 26.

101. **Xu B.** [Effect of acupuncture on the convalescence of meningioma removal.] *Zhongguo Zhongyiyao Xinxi Zazhi* [News Letters of Chinese Medicine], 1998, **5**(3):47 [in Chinese].

102. **Zhang LH et al.** A control study of scalp acupuncture in treating aphasia after acute cerebrovascular disease. *World Journal of Acupuncture-Moxibustion*, 1994, **4**(1):20 – 23.

103. **Lewith GT et al.** Acupuncture compared with placebo in post-herpetic pain. *Pain*, 1983, 17:361 – 368.

104. **Sukandar SD et al.** [Curing effect of acupuncture in post-herpetic neuralgia.] *Majalah Kedokteran Indonesia [Journal of the Indonesian Medical Association]*, 1995, 45(8): 456 – 461 [in Indonesian].

105. **Lin L.** Through puncture compared with traditional acupuncture in treating facial paralysis. *International Journal of Clinical Acupuncture*, 1997, 8(1):73–75.

106. **You FY et al.** [Observation of the effect of picking-out (blood-letting) acupuncture in the treatment of Bell's palsy.] *Shanghai Journal of Acupuncture and Moxibustion*, 1993, 12(2):74 [in Chinese].

107. **Liu XR.** [Observation of therapeutic effects of 66 cases of facial spasm treated with wrist-ankle acupuncture and body-acupuncture.] *Chinese Acupuncture and Moxibustion*, 1996, 16(4):192 [in Chinese].

108. **Frost EAM.** Acupuncture for the comatose patient. *American Journal of Acupuncture*, 1976, 4(1):45 – 48.

109. **Luo ZP et al.** [Clinical observation of ear-acupressure treatment of insomnia.] *Heilongjiang Journal of Traditional Chinese Medicine*, 1993, (1):45 – 48 [in Chinese].

110. **Zhang XF.** [Ear acupressure in the treatment of insomnia]. *Chinese Acupuncture and Moxibustion*, 1993, 13(6):297 – 298 [in Chinese].

111. **Chari P et al.** Acupuncture therapy in allergic rhinitis. *American Journal of Acupuncture*, 1988, 16(2):143 – 147.

112. **Huang YQ.** [Therapeutic effect of acupuncture treatment in 128 cases of hay fever.] *Chinese Acupuncture and Moxibustion*, 1990, 10(6):296 – 297 [in Chinese].

113. **Jin R et al.** [Clinical observation of 100 cases with allergic rhinitis treated by acupuncture.] *Chinese Acupuncture and Moxibustion*, 1989, 9(4):185 – 186 [in Chinese].

114. **Liu DX.** [Acupuncture at biqiu in the treatment of allergic rhinitis.] *Chinese Acupuncture and Moxibustion*, 1995, 15(6):293 [in Chinese].

115. **Yu JL et al.** [Effect of acupuncture treatment in 230 cases of allergic rhinitis.] *Chinese Acupuncture and Moxibustion*, 1994, 14(5):241 – 242 [in Chinese].

116. **Williamson L et al.** Hay fever treatment in general practice: a randomised controlled trial comparing standardised Western acupuncture with sham acupuncture. *Acupuncture-Medicine*, 1996, 14(1):6–10.

117. **Chen RH.** [Acupuncture treatment of 220 cases of acute tonsillitis.] *Chinese Acupuncture and Moxibustion*, 1987, 7(3):54 [in Chinese].

118. **Gunsberger M.** Acupuncture in the treatment of sore throat symptomatology. *American Journal of Chinese Medicine*, 1973, 1:337 – 340.

119. **Fung KP et al.** Attenuation of exercise-induced asthma by acupuncture. *Lancet*, 1986, 2:1419 – 1422.

120. **He YZ et al.** [Clinical observation of CO_2 laser acupuncture in the treatment of bronchial asthma.] *Chinese Acupuncture and Moxibustion, 1994, 14(1):13 – 16 [in Chinese].

121. **Tashkin DP et al.** Comparison of real and simulated acupuncture and isoproterenol in methacholine-induced asthma. *Annals of Allergy*, 1977, 39:379 – 387.

122. **Xie JP et al.** Observation of the specificity of points in electro-acupuncture treatment of asthma. *Chinese Acupuncture and Moxibustion*, 1996, 16(2):84 – 86 [in Chinese].

123. **Yu DC et al.** Effect of acupuncture on bronchial asthma. *Clinical Science and Molecular Medicine*, 1976, 51:503 – 509.

124. **Joshi YM.** Acupuncture in bronchial asthma. *Journal of the Association of Physicians of India,* 1992, **40**(5):327 – 331.

125. **Tandon MA et al.** Comparison of real and placebo acupuncture in histamine-induced asthma: a double-blind crossover study. *Chest,* 1989, 96:102 – 105.

126. **Batra YK et al.** Acupuncture in corticosteroid-dependent asthmatics. *American Journal of Acupuncture,* 1986, **14**(3):261 – 264.

127. **Jobst K et al.** Controlled trial of acupuncture for disabling breathlessness. *Lancet,* 1986, **2**:1416 – 1419.

128. **Xu PC et al.** Clinical observation of treatment of acute epigastralgia by puncturing liangqiu and weishu acupoints. *International Journal of Clinical Acupuncture,* 1991, **2**(2):127 – 130.

129. **Yu YM.** [Therapeutic effect and mechanism of needling ST36 in the treatment of epigastric pain.] *Shanghai Journal of Acupuncture and Moxibustion,* 1997, **16**(3):10 – 11 [in Chinese].

130. **Shi XL et al.** [Acupuncture treatment of gastrointestinal spasm.] *Chinese Acupuncture and Moxibustion,* 1995, **15**(4):192 [in Chinese].

131. **Zhang AL et al.** Clinical effect of acupuncture in the treatment of gastrokinetic disturbance. *World Journal of Acupuncture-Moxibustion,* 1996, **6**(1):3 – 8.

132. **Vickers AJ.** Can acupuncture have specific effects on health? A systematic review of acupuncture antiemesis trials. *Journal of the Royal Society of Medicine,* 1996, **89**(6): 303 – 311.

133. **Wu HG et al.** Preliminary study on therapeutic effects and immunologic mechanisms of herbal-moxibustion treatment of irritable bowel syndrome. *Chinese Acupuncture and Moxibustion,* 1996, **16**(2):43 – 45 [in Chinese].

134. **Wu HG et al.** [Therapeutic effect of herbal partition-moxibustion for chronic diarrhoea and its immunological mechanism.] *Journal of Traditional Chinese Medicine,* 1995, **36**(1):25 – 27 [in Chinese].

135. **Wang HH et al.** A study in the effectiveness of acupuncture analgesia for colonoscopic examination compared with conventional premedication. *American Journal of Acupuncture,* 1992, **20**:217 – 221.

136. **Wang HH et al.** A clinical study on physiological response in electroacupuncture analgesia and meperidine analgesia for colonoscopy. *American Journal of Chinese Medicine,* 1997, **25**(1):13–20.

137. **Diehl DL.** Acupuncture for gastrointestinal and hepatobiliary disorders. *Journal of Alternative and Complementary Medicine,* 1999, **5**(1):27–45.

138. **Zhao SD et al.** [Electro-acupuncture and magnesium sulphate in treatment of cholelithiasis—clinical observations on 522 cases and preliminary consideration of features.] *Chinese Medical Journal,* 1979, **59**(12):716 [in Chinese].

139. **Gong CM et al.** [Clinical study on regulatory action of combination of body acupuncture with auricular acupuncture on gallbladder motor function.] *Chinese Acupuncture and Moxibustion,* 1996, **16**(1):1 – 3 [in Chinese].

140. **Chen B et al.** [Clinical observation of moxibustion treatment of leukopenia caused by chemotherapy.] *Guo Yi Lun Tan* [Forum of Traditional Chinese Medicine], 1990, **5**(6):27 – 28 [in Chinese].

141. **Chen HL et al.** [Observation of the treatment of chemotherapy-induced leucocytopenia with acupuncture and moxibustion.] *Chinese Journal of Integrated Traditional and Western Medicine,* 1991, **11**(6):350 – 352 [in Chinese].

142. **Wang X.** [Effect of moxibustion in the treatment of chemotherapy-induced leukopenia.] [*Chinese Acupuncture and Moxibustion,* 1997, **17**(1):13 – 14 [in Chinese].

143. **Yin ZF et al.** [Therapeutic effect of acupuncture in the treatment of leucopenia induced by benzene.] *Jiangsu Journal of Traditional Chinese Medicine,* 1990, **11**(9)404 – 405 [in Chinese].

144. **Yin ZF et al.** Clinical approach to treatment of benzene-induced leucopenia with acupuncture. *World Journal of Acupuncture-Moxibustion*, 1992, **2**(3):15 – 18.

145. **He LY et al.** [Observation of therapeutic effect on 30 cases of puerperal retention of urine treated by acupuncture.] *Chinese Acupuncture and Moxibustion*, 1983, **3**(5):196 [in Chinese]

146. **Pan XW et al.** [Application of acupuncture therapy in traumatic urinary retention.] *Chinese Acupuncture and Moxibustion*, 1996, **16**(11):596 – 597 [in Chinese].

147. **Aydin S et al.** Acupuncture and hypnotic suggestions in the treatment of non-organic male sexual dysfunction. *Scandinavian Journal of Urology and Nephrology*, 1997, **31**(3):271–274.

148. **Shui HD.** [Acupuncture treatment of defective ejaculation.] *Chinese Acupuncture and Moxibustion*, 1986, **6**(1):19 [in Chinese].

149. **Luo YN et al.** Clinical research on treatment of chronic prostatitis with acupuncture. *World Journal of Acupuncture-Moxibustion*, 1994, **4**(3):7 – 14.

150. **Wang SY et al.** [The effect of acupuncture in lowering the urethral pressure of female urethral syndrome patients.] *Shanghai Journal of Acupuncture and Moxibustion*, 1997, **16**(2):4 – 6 [in Chinese].

151. **Zheng HT et al.** [Acupuncture treatment of female urethral syndrome.] *Chinese Acupuncture and Moxibustion*, 1997, **17**(12):719 – 721 [in Chinese].

152. **Aune A et al.** Acupuncture in the prophylaxis of recurrent lower urinary tract infection in adult women. *Scandinavian Journal of Primary Health Care*, 1998, **16**(1):37–39.

153. **Helms JM.** Acupuncture for the management of primary dysmenorrhea. *Obstetrics and Gynecology*, 1987, **69**:51 – 56.

154. **Shi XL et al.** [Acupuncture at SP 6 in the treatment of primary dysmenorrhoea.] *Chinese Acupuncture and Moxibustion*, 1994, **14**(5):241 – 242 [in Chinese].

155. **Li J et al.** [Treatment of 108 cases of premenstrual tension by head-acupuncture.] *Chinese Acupuncture and Moxibustion*, 1992, **12**(3):245 – 246 [in Chinese].

156. **Yu J et al.** [Relationship of hand temperature and blood β-endorphin immunoreactive substance with electroacupuncture induction of ovulation.] *Acupuncture Research*, 1986, **11**(2):86–90 [in Chinese].

157. **Chen BY.** Acupuncture normalized dysfunction of hypothalamic-pituitary-ovarian axis. *Acupuncture and Electro-Therapeutics Research*, 1997, **22**:97–108.

158. **Ji P et al.** [Clinical study on acupuncture treatment of infertility due to inflammatory obstruction of fallopian tube.] *Chinese Acupuncture and Moxibustion*, 1996, **16**(9):469 – 470 [in Chinese].

159. **Lin PC et al.** [Observation of the effect of acupuncture and oxytocin intravenous perfusion for expediting labour.] *Chinese Acupuncture and Moxibustion*, 1992, **12**(6):281 – 283 [in Chinese].

160. **Ma WZ et al.** [Clinical observation of the influence of puncturing different points on the whole stage of labour.] *Chinese Acupuncture and Moxibustion*, 1995, **15**(3):130 – 131 [in Chinese].

161. **Yu XZ et al.** [Observation of hastening of parturition and induction of labour with acupuncture.] *Chinese Journal of Integrated Traditional and Western Medicine*, 1981, **1**(1):12 – 15 [in Chinese].

162. **Dundee JW et al.** PC 6 acupressure reduces morning sickness. *Journal of the Royal Society of Medicine*, 1988, **81**(8):456 – 457.

163. **Fan YJ.** Observation of the therapeutic effect of moxibustion for treatment of pregnant vomiting. *World Journal of Acupuncture-Moxibustion*, 1995, **5**(4):31 – 33.

164. **Cardini F et al.** Moxibustion for correction of breech presentation: a randomized controlled trial. *Journal of the American Medical Association*, 1998, **280**(18):1580–1584.

165. **Li GR et al.** [Correction of abnormal foetal position by moxibustion in 74 cases.] *Journal of .Acupuncture-Moxibustion*, 1990, **30**(3):11 [in Chinese].

166. **Li Q.** Clinical observation of correcting malposition of fetus by electro-acupuncture. *Journal of Traditional Chinese Medicine*, 1996, **16**(4):260–262.

167. **Qin GF et al.** [Correction of abnormal foetal position by ear point pressure—a report of 413 cases.] *China Journal of Traditional Chinese Medicine*, 1989, **30**(6):350–352 [in Chinese].

168. **Hu XC et al.** [The influence of acupuncture on blood prolactin level in women with deficient lactation.] *Shanghai Journal of Traditional Chinese Medicine*, 1958, (12):557–558 [in Chinese].

169. **Chandra A et al.** [The influences of acupuncture on breast feeding production.] *Cermin Dunia Kedokteran*, 1995, (105):33 ‐ 37 [in Indonesian].

170. **Guo JS.** [Clinical observation of 150 cases of primary hypotension treated by vaccaria seeds pressed on ear points.] *Chinese Acupuncture and Moxibustion*, 1992, **12**(6):295 ‐ 296 [in Chinese].

171. **Yu L et al.** [Treatment of 180 cases of hypotension with G20 needling.] *Shanghai Journal of Acupuncture and Moxibustion*, 1998, **17**(4):8 [in Chinese].

172. **Dan Y.** [Assessment of acupuncture treatment of hypertension by ambulatory blood pressure monitoring.] *Chinese Journal of Integrated Traditional and Western Medicine*, 1998, **18**(1):26–27 [in Chinese].

173. **Iurenev AP et al.** [Use of various non-pharmacological methods in the treatment of patients in the early stages of arterial hypertension.] *Terapevticheskii Arkhiv*, 1988, **60**(1):123 ‐ 126 [in Russian].

174. **Wu CX et al.** Scalp acupuncture in treating hypertension in the elderly. *International Journal of Clinical Acupuncture*, 1997, **8**(3):281–284.

175. **Yu P et al.** Clinical study on auricular pressure treatment of primary hypertension. *International Journal of Clinical Acupuncture*, 1991, **2**(1):37 ‐ 40.

176. **Zhou RX et al.** [The hypotensive effect of ear acupressure—an analysis of 274 cases.] *China Journal of Traditional Chinese Medicine*, 1990, **30**(2):99 ‐ 100 [in Chinese]

177. **Cai QC et al.** [The regulatory effects of acupuncture on blood pressure and serum nitrogen monoxide levels in patients with hypertension.] *Chinese Acupuncture and Moxibustion*, 1998, **18**(1):9–11 [in Chinese].

178. **Zhou YM.** [Observation of the therapeutic effect of 30 cases of cardiac neurosis treated with acupuncture at renying.] *Chinese Acupuncture and Moxibustion*, 1992, **12**(2):30 ‐ 32 [in Chinese].

179. **Ballegaard S.** Acupuncture and the cardiovascular system: a scientific challenge. *Acupuncture-Medicine*, 1998, **16**(1):2–9.

180. **Ballegaard S et al.** Acupuncture in severe, stable angina pectoris: a randomized trial. *Acta Medica Scandinavica*, 1986, **220**(4):307 ‐ 313.

181. **Ballegaard S et al.** Effects of acupuncture in moderate, stable angina pectoris: a controlled study. *Journal of Internal Medicine*, 1990, **227**(1):25 ‐ 30.

182. **Dai JY et al.** [Clinical observation of ear acupuncture at point heart in the treatment of coronary heart disease.] *Journal of Traditional Chinese Medicine*, 1995, **36**(11):664 ‐ 665 [in Chinese].

183. **Cheng BA.** [Clinical observation of ear acupressure treatment in 50 cases of angina pectoris.] *Chinese Acupuncture and Moxibustion*, 1995, **15**(2):74 ‐ 75 [in Chinese].

184. **Mao XR et al.** Effects of acupuncture on angina pectoris, ECG and blood lipids of patients with coronary heart disease. *World Journal of Acupuncture-Moxibustion*, 1993, **3**(4):15 ‐ 19.

185. **Zhou XQ et al.** [Influence of acupuncture on the calibre of coronary artery in coronary heart disease.] *Journal of the Hunan College of Traditional Chinese Medicine*, 1990, **10**(3):166–167 [in Chinese].

186. **Xue SM et al.** Effects of acupuncture on the left ventricular diastolic function in patients with coronary heart disease. *World Journal of Acupuncture-Moxibustion*, 1992, **2**(2):10.

187. **Ho FM et al.** Effect of acupuncture at nei-kuan on left ventricular function in patients with coronary artery disease. *American Journal of Chinese Medicine*, 1999, **27**(2):149–156.

188. **Hu NK et al.** [Acupuncture at neiguan causes haemorrheological improvement in patients with coronary heart disease.] *Zhong Xi Yi Jiehe Shiyong Linchuang Jijiu [Clinical Emergency by Integrated Chinese and Western Medicine]*, 1997, **4**(5):206–207 [in Chinese].

189. **Hou DF et al.** [Clinical observation of therapeutic effect of baihui (GV20)-yintang (EX‑HN3) electro-acupuncture in 30 cases of post-apoplectic depression.] *Chinese Acupuncture and Moxibustion*, 1996, **16**(8):432‑433 [in Chinese].

190. **Li CD et al.** Treating post-stroke depression with "antidepressive" acupuncture therapy: A clinical study of 21 cases. *International Journal of Clinical Acupuncture*, 1994, **5**(4):389‑393.

191. **Luo HC et al.** Electro-acupuncture vs amitriptyline in the treatment of depressive states. *Journal of Traditional Chinese Medicine*, 1985, **5**(1):3–8.

192. **Luo HC et al.** [Clinical observation of electro-acupuncture on 133 patients with depression in comparison with tricyclic amytriptyline.] *Chinese Journal of Integrated Traditional and Western Medicine*, 1988, **8**(2):77‑80 [in Chinese].

193. **Yang X.** Clinical observation of needling extrameridian points in treating mental depression. *Journal of Traditional Chinese Medicine*, 1994, **14**:14‑18.

194. **Zhang B et al.** A control study of clinical therapeutic effects of laser-acupuncture on depressive neurosis. *World Journal of Acupuncture-Moxibustion*, 1996, **6**(2):12‑17.

195. **Jia YK et al.** [Treatment of schizophrenia with helium-neon laser irradiation at acupoints.] *Chinese Acupuncture and Moxibustion*, 1986, **6**(1):19–21 [in Chinese].

196. **Que YT et al.** [Observation of 111 cases of competition stress syndrome treated with auriculo-pressure therapy.] *Chinese Acupuncture and Moxibustion*, 1986, **6**(2):57 [in Chinese].

197. **Wen HL et al.** Treatment of drug addiction by acupuncture and electrical stimulation. *Asian Journal of Medicine*, 1993, **9**:138‑141.

198. **Culliton RD et al.** Overview of substance abuse acupuncture treatment research. *Journal of Alternative and Complementary Medicine*, 1996, **2**(1):149‑159.

199. **Bullock ML et al.** Auricular acupuncture in the treatment of cocaine abuse: a study of efficacy and dosing. *Journal of Substance Abuse Treatment*, 1999, **16**(1):31–38.

200. **Cai Z et al.** [Acupuncture treatment in the late stage of addiction abstinence.] *Jiangsu Journal of Traditional Chinese Medicine*, 1998, **19**(12):35 [in Chinese].

201. **Margolin A et al.** Acupuncture for the treatment of cocaine dependence in methadone-maintained patients. *American Journal of Addiction*, 1993, **2**(3):194‑201.

202. **Washburn AM et al.** Acupuncture heroin detoxification: a single-blind clinical trial. *Journal of Substance Abuse Treatment*, 1993, **10**:345‑351.

203. **Clavel F et al.** [A study of various smoking cessation programs based on close to 1000 volunteers recruited from the general population: 1-month results.] *Revue Epidemiologique de Santé Publique*, 1990, **38**(2):133‑138 [in French].

204. **Fang YA.** [Clinical study on giving up smoking with acupuncture.] *Shanghai Journal of Acupuncture and Moxibustion*, 1983, **2**(2):30‑31 [in Chinese].

205. **He D et al.** Effects of acupuncture on smoking cessation or reduction for motivated smokers. *Preventive Medicine*, 1997, **26**(2):208–214.

206. **Waite NR et al.** A single-blind, placebo-controlled trial of a simple acupuncture treatment in the cessation of smoking. *British Journal off General Practice*, 1998, **48**(433):1487–1490.

207. **White AR et al.** Randomized trial of acupuncture for nicotine withdrawal symptoms. *Archives of Internal Medicine,* 1998, **158**(20):2251–2255.

208. **White AR et al.** [Smoking cessation with acupuncture? A 'best evidence synthesis']. *Forschende Komplimentarmedizin,* 1997, **4**(2):102–105 [in German].

209. **Bullock ML et al.** Controlled trial of acupuncture for severe recidivist alcoholism. *Lancet,* 1990, **335**:20 – 21.

210. **Bullock ML et al.** Acupuncture treatment of alcoholic recidivism: a pilot study. *American Journal of Acupuncture,* 1987, **15**(4):313–320.

211. **Bullock ML et al.** Controlled trial of acupuncture for severe recidivist alcoholism. *Lancet,* 1989, 1:1435 – 1439.

212. **Thorer H et al.** Acupuncture after alcohol consumption: a sham controlled assessment. *Acupuncture-Medicine,* 1996, 14(2):63–67.

213. **Li YQ et al.** Swift needling of zusanli and changqiang in treating infantile diarrhea. *International Journal of Clinical Acupuncture,* 1997, **8**(2):187–189.

214. **Yang ZW.** [Treatment of 100 cases of infantile diarrhoea by acupuncture.] *Shanghai Journal of Acupuncture and Moxibustion,* 1998, **17**(6):11. [in Chinese].

215. **He JX et al.** [Therapeutic effect of acupuncture at LI 4 in the treatment of infantile convulsion due to high fever.] *Zhong Xi Yi Jiehe Shiyong Linchuang Jijiu* [Clinical Emergency by Integrated Chinese and Western Medicine], 1997, **4**(8):360 – 361 [in Chinese].

216. **Jin MZ.** [Acupuncture plus auricular acupressure treatment of 30 cases of Gilles de la Tourette's syndrome.] *Guangming Traditional Chinese Medicine,* 1998, **78**(5):23 – 24 [in Chinese].

217. **Tian LD et al.** [Observation of therapeutic effects of 68 cases of Gilles de la Tourette's syndrome in children treated with acupuncture.] *Chinese Acupuncture and Moxibustion,* 1996, **16**(9):483 – 484 [in Chinese].

218. **Wang CH et al.** [Clinical study on acupuncture treatment of sudden deafness.] *Acupuncture Research,* 1998, **23**(1):5 – 7 [in Chinese].

219. **Zhang ZF et al.** [Clinical study on acupuncture treatment of acute attack of Ménière's syndrome.] *Shanghai Journal of Acupuncture and Moxibustion,* 1983, **2**(4):28 [in Chinese].

220. **Jin XQ et al.** [Clinical observation of 35 cases of subjective tinnitus treated with acupuncture.] *Zhejiang Journal of Traditional Chinese Medicine,* 1998, **33**(3):118 [in Chinese].

221. **Vilholm OJ et al.** Effect of traditional Chinese acupuncture on severe tinnitus: a double-blind, placebo-controlled clinical investigation with open therapeutic control. *British Journal of Audiology,* 1998, **32**(3):197–204.

222. **Mekhamer A et al.** Experience with unexplained otalgia. *Pain,* 1987, (Suppl.):361.

223. **Lang BX et al.** [Clinical observation of the therapeutic effect of ear acupuncture in treating simple epistaxis.] *Chinese Acupuncture and Moxibustion,* 1995, **15**(2):76 – 77 [in Chinese].

224. **Luan YH et al.** [Clinical observation of 60 cases of chloasma treated with auricular acupuncture and acupressure.] *Chinese Acupuncture and Moxibustion,* 1996, **16**(9):485 – 486 [in Chinese].

225. **Chen BZ et al.** Comparative observation of the curative effects of herpes zoster treated by type JI He-Ne laser and polyinosinic acid. *World Journal of Acupuncture-Moxibustion,* 1994, **4**(2):29 – 31.

226. **Lunderberg T et al.** Effect of acupuncture on experimentally induced itch. *British Journal of Dermatology,* 1987, **17**:771 – 777.

227. **Huang BS et al.** [Treatment of 60 cases of neurodermatitis with three-step seven-star needling therapy.] *Journal of Guiyang Chinese Medical College,* 1998, **20**(2):35–36 [in Chinese].

228. **Li HQ et al.** [Acupuncture treatment in 42 cases of acne vulgaris.] *Chinese Acupuncture and Moxibustion*, 1998, **18**(3):166 [in Chinese].

229. **Wang J et al.** [Auriculo-acupuncture treatment of 32 cases of facial acne vulgaris.] *Shanghai Journal of Acupuncture and Moxibustion*, 1997, **16**(3):25 [in Chinese].

230. **Dang W et al.** [Clinical study on acupuncture treatment of pain caused by stomach cancer.] *Journal of Traditional Chinese Medicine*, 1995, **36**(5):277 ‒ 280 [in Chinese].

231. **Dan Y et al.** [Clinical study on analgesic effect of acupuncture on carcinomatous pain.] *Chinese Acupuncture and Moxibustion*, 1998, **18**(1):17 ‒ 18 [in Chinese].

232. **Chen GP et al.** [Observation of therapeutic effects of acupuncture in 44 cases with gastrointestinal reaction induced by radiotherapy and chemotherapy.] *Chinese Acupuncture and Moxibustion*, 1996, **16**(7):359 ‒ 360 [in Chinese].

233. **Dundee JW et al.** Acupuncture to prevent cisplatin-associated vomiting. *Lancet*, 1987, **1**:1083.

234. **Li H et al.** Clinical study on acupuncture treatment of side reactions of radiotherapy and chemotherapy for malignant tumour. *World Journal of Acupuncture-Moxibustion*, 1998, **8**(2):8 ‒ 12.

235. **Liu A et al.** [Clinical research on attenuating chemotherapeutic toxicity by acupoint stimulation therapy.] *Shanghai Journal of Acupuncture and Moxibustion*, 1998, **17**(6):8 ‒ 9 [in Chinese].

236. **Wang SZ et al.** [Clinical study on acupuncture control of gastrointestinal reactions to chemotherapy.] *Chinese Acupuncture and Moxibustion*, 1997, **17**(1):17 ‒ 18 [in Chinese].

237. **Xia YQ et al.** [Acupuncture treatment of reactions due to radiotherapy in patients with malignant tumour.] *Chinese Acupuncture and Moxibustion*, 1984, **4**(6):6 ‒ 8 [in Chinese].

238. **Richards D et al.** Stimulation of auricular acupuncture points in weight loss. *Australian Family Physician*, 1998, **27**(S2):S73–77.

239. **Wang H.** Clinical analysis on treatment of 40 cases of hyperlipemia with point-injection of radix salviae miltiorrhizae injection. *World Journal of Acupuncture-Moxibustion*, 1998, **8**(4):20 ‒ 22.

240. **Kang SY et al.** [Clinical investigation of the treatment of diabetes mellitus with timing acupuncture.] *Chinese Acupuncture and Moxibustion*, 1995, **15**(1):6 ‒ 8 [in Chinese].

241. **Latief R.** The effect of san yin ciao point on hyperglycemia of non-insulin-dependent diabetes mellitus. *Cermin Dumia Kedokteran*, 1987, (44):20 ‒ 23 [in Indonesian].

242. **Xiong DZ et al.** [Observation of the therapeutic effect of acupuncture in the treatment of drug-induced sialorrhea.] *Chinese Acupuncture and Moxibustion*, 1993, **13**(3):137 ‒ 138 [in Chinese].

243. **List T et al.** The effect of acupuncture in the treatment of patients with primary Sjögren's syndrome: a controlled study. *Acta Odontologica Scandinavica*, 1998, **56**(2):95–99.

244. **Appiah R et al.** Treatment of primary Raynaud's syndrome with traditional Chinese acupuncture. *Journal of Internal Medicine*, 1997, **241**(2):119–124.

245. **Ma RH et al.** [Clinical observation of acupuncture treatment in polycystic ovary syndrome.] *Chinese Acupuncture and Moxibustion*, 1996, **16**(11):602 ‒ 623 [in Chinese].

246. **Yang XT.** [Observation of 108 cases of Tietze's syndrome treated with short needling plus cupping.] *Chinese Acupuncture and Moxibustion*, 1997, **17**(7):435 ‒ 436 [in Chinese].

247. **Wolkenstein E, Horak F.** A statistical evaluation of the protective effect of acupuncture against allergen-provoked rhinitis. *Deutsche Zeitschrift für Akupunktur,* 1993, **36**(6):132 – 137.

248. **Biernacki W et al.** Acupuncture in treatment of stable asthma. *Respiratory Medicine,* 1998, **92**(9):1143–1145.

249. **Ding ZS.** [Observation of therapeutic effect of 120 cases of bulbar paralysis treated with acupuncture.] *Chinese Acupuncture and Moxibustion,* 1996, **16**(3):128 – 129 [in Chinese].

250. **Cai ZM.** [The effect of acupuncture and auricular acupressure on colour discrimination.] *Chinese Acupuncture and Moxibustion,* 1998, **18**(9):521 – 522 [in Chinese].

251. **Ma RZ et al.** Clinical observation and study of mechanisms of acupuncture treatment of coronary heart disease. *World Journal of Acupuncture-Moxibustion,* 1997, **7**(1):3 – 8.

252. **Ding J et al.** Comparative observation of curative effects of postoperative symptoms of the closed craniocerebral injury treated by acupuncture. *World Journal of Acupuncture-Moxibustion,* 1997, **7**(3):26 – 28.

253. **Clavel F et al.** Helping people to stop smoking: randomized comparison of groups being treated with acupuncture and nicotine gum with control group. *British Medical Journal,* 1985, **291**:1538 – 1539.

254. **Luo H et al.** Clinical research on the therapeutic effect of the electroacupuncture treatment in patients with depression. *Psychiatry and Clinical Neurosciences,* 1998, **52** (Suppl.): S338–S340.

255. **Liu ZS et al.** [Clinical study on acupuncture treatment of dysphagia in pseudobulbar paralysis.] *New Traditional Chinese Medicine,* 1998, **30**(3):24 – 25. [in Chinese].

256. **Ma RH et al.** [Clinical observation of 56 cases of hypo-ovarianism treated with acupuncture.] *Chinese Acupuncture and Moxibustion,* 1997, **17**(7):395 – 396 [in Chinese].

257. **Tian LT et al.** [Clinical observation of 100 children of hypophrenia treated mainly with acupuncture.] *Chinese Acupuncture and Moxibustion,* 1996, **16**(6):292 – 293 [in Chinese].

258. **De Aloysio D, Penacchioni P.** Morning sickness control in early pregnancy by eiguan point acupressure. *Obstetrics and Gynecology,* 1992 **80**(5): 852–854.

259. **Bayreuther J, Lewith GT, Pickering R.** A double-blind cross-over study to evaluate the effectiveness of acupressure at pericardium 6 (P6) in the treatment of early morning sickness (EMS). *Complementary Therapies in Medicine,* 1994, **2**:70–76.

260. **Dundee JW et al.** Traditional Chinese acupuncture: a potentially useful antiemetic? *British Medical Journal,* 1986, **293**:383 – 384.

261. **Ghaly RG et al.** A comparison of manual needling with electrical stimulation and commonly used antiemetics. *Anaesthesia,* 1987, **45**:1108 – 1110.

262. **Weightman WM et al.** Traditional Chinese acupuncture as an antiemetic. *British Medical Journal,* 1987, **295**(6610):1379–1380.

263. **Dundee JW et al.** Acupuncture prophylaxis of cancer chemotherapy-induced sickness. *Journal of the Royal Society of Medicine,* 1989, **82**:268–271.

264. **Barsoum G et al.** Postoperative nausea is relieved by acupressure. *Journal of the Royal Society of Medicine,* 1990, **83**(2):86 – 89.

265. **Ho RT et al.** Electro-acupuncture and postoperative emesis. *Anaesthesia,* 1990, **45**:327 – 329.

266. **Ho CM et al.** Effect of PC 6 acupressure on prevention of nausea and vomiting after epidural morphine for post-cesarean section pain relief. *Acta Anaesthesiologica Scandinavica,* 1996, **40**(3):372 – 375.

267. Andrzejowski J et al. Semi-permanent acupuncture needles in the prevention of postoperative nausea and vomiting. *Acupuncture-Medicine*, 1996, **14**(2):68–70.

268. McConaghy P et al. Acupuncture in the management of postoperative nausea and vomiting in patients receiving morphine via a patient-controlled analgesia system. *Acupuncture-Medicine*, 1996, **14**(1):2–5.

269. Schwager KL et al. Acupuncture and postoperative vomiting in day-stay paediatric patients. *Anaesthesia and Intensive Care*, 1996, **24**(6):674–677.

270. Liu SX et al. Magnetotherapy of neiguan in preventing vomiting induced by cisplatin. *International Journal of Clinical Acupuncture*, 1997, **8**(1):39–41.

271 Al-Sadi M et al. Acupuncture in the prevention of postoperative nausea and vomiting. *Anaesthesia*, 1997, **52**(7):658–661.

272. Stein DJ et al. Acupressure versus intravenous metoclopramide to prevent nausea and vomiting during spinal anesthesia for cesarean section. *Anesthesia and Analgesia*, 1997, **84**(2):342–345.

273. Schlager A et al. Laser stimulation of acupuncture point P6 reduces postoperative vomiting in children undergoing strabismus surgery. *British Journal of Anaesthesia*, 1998, **8**(4):529–532.

274. Chu YC et al. Effect of BL10 (tianzhu), BL11 (dazhu) and GB34 (yanglingquan) acuplaster for prevention of vomiting after strabismus surgery in children. *Acta Anaesthesiologica Sinica*, 1998, **36**(1):11–16.

275. Alkaissi A et al. Effect and placebo effect of acupressure (P6) on nausea and vomiting after outpatient gynaecological surgery. *Acta Anaesthesiologica Scandinavica*, 1999, **43**(3):270–274.

276. Shenkman Z et al. Acupressure-acupuncture antiemetic prophylaxis in children undergoing tonsillectomy. *Anesthesiology*, 1999, **90**(5):1311–1316.

277. Cheng PT et al. A therapeutic trial of acupuncture in neurogenic bladder of spinal cord injured patients—a preliminary report. *Spinal Cord*, 1998, **36**(7):476–480.

278. Felhendler D et al. Pressure on acupoints decreases postoperative pain. *Clinical Journal of Pain*, 1996, **12**(4):326–329.

279. Zou M et al. [Observation of therapeutic effects of combined treatment of ginger moxibustion and acupoint-injection in 30 cases of chronic pulmonary heart disease.] *Chinese Acupuncture and Moxibustion*, 1998, **18**(7):389–390 [in Chinese].

280. Kho KH. The impact of acupuncture on pain in patients with reflex sympathetic dystrophy. *Pain-Clinic*, 1995, **8**(1):59–61.

281. Yu DF et al. [Acupuncture treatment in 86 cases of central serous retinopathy.] *Chinese Acupuncture and Moxibustion*, 1997, **17**(5):273–274 [in Chinese].

282. Zhang B et al. [Controlled study of clinical effect of computer controlled electro-acupuncture in the treatment of schizophrenia.] *Chinese Acupuncture and Moxibustion*, 1994, **14**(1):17–20 [in Chinese].

283. Yu CQ et al. [Treatment of simple obesity in children with photo-acupuncture.] *Chinese Journal of Integrated Traditional and Western Medicine*, 1998, **18**(6):348–350 [in Chinese].

284. Chen Y et al. Observation of the time-effect of acupuncture in improving small airway function. *World Journal of Acupuncture-Moxibustion*, 1997, **7**(2):26–28.

285. Santiesteban AJ. Comparison of electro-acupuncture and selected physical therapy for acute spine pain. *American Journal of Acupuncture*, 1984, **12**(3):257–261.

286. Wu QF. 100 cases of stiff neck treated by contralateral acupuncture. *International Journal of Clinical Acupuncture*, 1997, **8**(4):427–429.

287. Zou XC et al. [Comparative study of cerebral infarction with acupuncture on six acupoints of yang meridian and calan tablets.] *Chinese Journal of Integrated Traditional and Western Medicine*, 1990, **10**(4):199–202 [in Chinese].

288. **Raustia AM et al.** Acupuncture compared with stomatognathic treatment for temporomandibular joint dysfunction. *Journal of Prosthetic Dentistry*, 1986, **56**(5):616 – 623.

289. **Ma S et al.** [Observation of combined acupuncture and moxibustion treatment of 60 cases of ulcerative colitis.] *Chinese Acupuncture and Moxibustion*, 1997, **17**(5):275 – 276 [in Chinese].

290. **Lai XS.** [Therapeutic effect of acupuncture in the treatment of senile vascular dementia.] *Chinese Acupuncture and Moxibustion*, 1997, **17**(4):201 – 202 [in Chinese].

291. **Liu J et al.** [Clinical study on treatment of vascular dementia by electroacupuncture of scalp acupoints.] *Chinese Acupuncture and Moxibustion*, 1998, **18**(4):197 – 200 [in Chinese].

292. **Jiang GH et al.** [Controlled observation of electro-acupuncture treatment of vascular dementia.] *Bulletin of Gaungzhou Traditional Chinese Medicine University*, 1998, **15**(2):110 – 112 [in Chinese].

293. **Wang LQ.** [A comparative study on acupuncture treatment of viral encephalitis in children.] *Chinese Acupuncture and Moxibustion*, 1998, **18**(7):397 – 398 [in Chinese].